Living Well with MS

Also by David L. Carroll

Living with Parkinson's
When Your Loved One Has Alzheimer's

Living Well with MS

A GUIDE FOR PATIENT, CAREGIVER, AND FAMILY

DAVID L. CARROLL

JON DUDLEY DORMAN, M.D.

HarperPerennial
A Division of HarperCollinsPublishers

FIRST EDITION

Designed by Alma Orenstein

Library of Congress Cataloging-in-Publication Data
Carroll, David L.
    Living well with MS : a guide for patient, caregiver, and family /
by David L. Carroll & Jon Dudley Dorman, M.D.
        p.   cm.
    Includes bibliographical references and index.
    ISBN 0-06-096980-6
    1. Multiple sclerosis—Popular works.   I. Dorman, Jon.
    II. Title.
RC377.C33   1993   92-53396
616.8'34—dc20

93 94 95 96 97 CC/RRD 10 9 8 7 6 5 4 3 2 1

Contents

Acknowledgments

The authors would like to thank the following for their help in making this book possible: Gina Marie DeSantis, Tracy Ellis, Mary Stamps, Dick Runk, Anita, Louise Marie Leigh, Donna Meade, Binny Farthing, Lester Dale Runyon, Ben Meeker, Leslie MacDonald, Mary Beth Markady, Jim Glinder, Richard Emilio, Nancy Schwartz, Jennifer Richardson, Laura Smith, Bill La Seur, Sunny Turner, Stacy Little, Ed Stamolla.

Special thanks go to Doctor Joseph Herbert for his precious time and valuable medical information; also to Mary Nishamoto for her expert input on several of the physical therapy sections included. Gratitude as well to Janet Gray and Margaret Knowland of Helen Hayes Hospital in Haverstraw, New York; to Dr. Della Williams, Dr. Lex Marcell, Billy Endelman, and Phil Stubbs.

Living Well with MS

1

All About
Multiple Sclerosis

FIRST THOUGHTS

Between a quarter- and a half-million persons in the United States today have multiple sclerosis. The first question that is asked by a majority of them when newly diagnosed by a physician is: "Will I die from this disease? Is it fatal?"

The answer is a definite no.

Multiple sclerosis, or MS as it is more commonly called, is not classified as a fatal ailment. Most patients live out the normal course of their lives, and the life-expectancy rate of an MS person is only slightly less than that of the national average. In the most severe cases it is possible that complications caused by symptoms can eventually lead to death; but, generally speaking, this is rare. MS is a disease that you can live with.

The second most common question that doctors hear immediately after a diagnosis is: "Is there a cure?"

Unfortunately, no.

Chemical medications do exist which will keep the disease under control in many instances, and which will palliate its symptoms. As yet, however—and though there are literally hundreds of claims, some within the margins of orthodoxy, some not—no one has yet produced accepted medical evidence that any form of chemotherapy, arsenic treatments, surgery, vaccine, diet, enzymes, ultrasound, chelation, dental therapy, megavitamin regimes, snake venom, sitz baths, or any others on the long list of candidates in any way cures this disorder.

The third thing patients want to know most commonly is: "How much will this disease affect my day-to-day functioning?"

Here the answer is less cut-and-dried, for at the very heart of this strange disorder is a profound unpredictability. Some people, for example, have MS all their lives and are rarely bothered by it. Others develop extremely serious symptoms and are wheelchair or bedbound within a year after the onset. A few never even know they have it.

A majority of patients, however, experience either a "relapsing-remitting" or a "relapsing-progressive" form of the disease, in which symptoms tend to come and go, leaving patients with stretches of time in which they suffer some discomforts but are able to live relatively normal lives.

One study shows, for example, that after twenty-five years, 65 percent of MS sufferers are still able to walk, talk, and manage the affairs of their daily lives in an efficient way. Such persons take precautions, of course, many of which we will discuss in this book. They tire easily. They may use canes when they walk to the corner store, or wear braces on their legs when they go out. They may not be able to ski or bungee jump, or do certain of the things that they did before they became sick. But they manage. MS in most cases is a manageable disease. A quote from the National Multiple Sclerosis Society's pamphlet *Living with MS* is apropos in this regard:

> The public image of MS is overly negative. MS is commonly associated with people in wheelchairs since those are the easily recognizable cases. The facts, however, reveal that most MS patients do not require wheelchairs. Many are only mildly incapacitated, and there are others who have no physically disabling symptoms at all. These people are often lost

to medical follow-up, and their mild cases are not reflected adequately by statistics. You will no doubt hear stories of people suffering the most severe cases of MS. Try to avoid making comparisons between yourself and other MS patients; every case is unique and unpredictable.*

A fourth question often comes up: "Is the disease contagious? Are other members of my family at risk?"

Here a flat no. There is no demonstrable evidence to show that multiple sclerosis can be passed on from one human being to another. Studies of married couples of whom one spouse has MS, for example, show conclusively that there is no increase in risk for the healthy partner. Within families in which one child has the disease there is a slight increase in incidence for siblings, but all available evidence indicates that this is due to genetics rather than contagion.

The last question frequently asked in the examining room is: "Will I experience much pain?"

Here again there are no sure answers, though the odds are heavily on a patient's side. Most persons with MS suffer various degrees of discomfort, but only a few complain of severe pain. In many cases, this pain can be relieved by medications. In some cases it can be fully eradicated.

One final fact to note about MS before we move on is that it is an entirely modern disease. At the end of the eighteenth century it was apparently unknown among the general population, and cases did not begin to appear on a regular basis until the middle of the 1800s.

While some researchers claim that the disease did, in fact, exist in earlier times but went undiagnosed, early medical reports do not back up this theory, and there is a conspicuous lack of historical symptom descriptions that in any way resemble those of MS.

Why this is so is difficult to say. It would seem at first that the answer is obvious: some by-product of the modern, industrial world attacks the nervous system and causes the disease. Sounds plausible. As yet, however, there is little evidence to demonstrate

*Lynn Wasserman, *Living with MS: A Practical Guide,* National Multiple Sclerosis Society, 1978.

a traceable relationship between MS and chemical or industrial wastes. Many studies have been made through the years focusing on the possible role of practically every type of toxin and pollutant: toxins in the water, in the air, in the soil, in food. None have shown any correlation with the development of MS.

For the time being, therefore, we must satisfy ourselves with the disconcerting reality that MS is an unpredictable and elusive ailment that comes and goes, and that so far defies all attempts at fully understanding its cause.

With these facts in mind, let's have a closer look at the particulars of the disease.

THE DISEASE PROCESS

Multiple sclerosis is a chronic neurological disorder of the central nervous system (CNS)—the brain and the spinal cord. There are several types of cells that compose this system. For our purposes the most important are the nerve cells.

Tiny, tree-shaped marvels of nature, human nerve cells are composed of delicate fibers known as *axons* that extend throughout the body in gossamer networks that crisscross in staggeringly complex patterns, carrying crucial neurological messages to different parts of the body, and ultimately connecting the central nervous system to other vital organs such as the sensorium (the eyes, ears, nose, etc.), the heart, lungs, and practically every other part of the human machine.

Nerve fibers are composed of highly sensitive tissues, and they require a special housing to protect them. Nature has thus threaded them through the body in a layered casing of white fatty tissue known as *myelin sheaths*. These sheaths insulate the fibers from abuse, and help quicken the transfer of nerve impulses along them.

For reasons presently unknown (more on the causes of MS below) small patches on these myelin sheaths are attacked and stripped in a way that is roughly analogous to what happens when an electrician peels a small piece of plastic insulation off an electric wire. Soon thereafter star-shaped neuroglial cells known as *oligo-dendrocytes* and *astrocytes* arrive on the scene to repair the damaged sites, but during this rebuilding process they cause scar tissue, known as *gliotic plaques,* to form.

These plaques become hard and sclerotic—a sclerosis is a thickening or hardening of cellular tissue—and then begin to interfere with or obstruct the flow of nerve impulses that pass along the nerve cells.

Normally, for example, nerve impulses travel along axonal pathways at around 225 miles an hour. When a section of myelin sheath is destroyed, however, nerve impulses are slowed down to half that speed or even less. This means that command messages sent, say, from the brain to the bladder telling the bladder to release urine do not arrive at their normal speed, and often become garbled or confused in the transmission. The bladder, consequently, does not release its urine on cue, and an enlarged bladder with concomitant dribbling and incontinence results.

If a sclerotic plaque is small, about the size of a pinhole, the disturbances it produces may affect only a single function of the body. If large, an inch or longer, it may disturb several functions at once. If a plaque heals and then another forms elsewhere in the CNS, the type of symptom produced will change, along with its location in the body. If several plaques are active at the same time they will produce multiple disturbances.

The symptoms produced by demyelination correspond to the particular areas of the nervous system that are attacked and demyelinated. For example, if a sclerotic plaque forms on the optic nerve, it will in all likelihood interfere with the flow of vision messages to the brain, and hence with one's ability to see properly. If it is on the spinal cord it may produce spasticity or bladder dysfunction. If one or more plaques are in the brain, fatigue may occur along with slurred speech, dizziness, and/or muscle weakness in the arms. The type of symptoms produced, in other words, depends on 1) the size of the sclerotic plaque; 2) where in the central nervous system the plaque situates itself; 3) how many of these plaques are present at a given time.

It is this very fact that MS plaques can be disseminated in so many different places along the central nervous system, and that several plaques may be active at one time, that earns the disease the name of "multiple" sclerosis, i.e., many scars in many places. An alternative name, used more commonly in England than the United States, is "disseminated sclerosis."

Course of Development

Although multiple sclerosis is considered to be a progressive disease, progression does not inevitably occur. Note:

1. Statistically speaking, approximately 20 percent of MS patients suffer plaque formation and demyelination, recover, and then never experience a recurrence. The origins of the disease may, perhaps, remain hidden within their systems, but none of its symptoms ever return.

2. Thirty percent of MS patients experience one or several episodes of MS symptoms, which then pass into remission and do not reappear again for years or even decades. This is the relapsing-remitting form of the disease.

3. Forty percent of MS patients experience a slow and steady progression of symptoms through the years, with an increasing number of flareups occurring as time passes. This form is known as relapsing-progressing.

4. Ten percent of patients experience multiple disturbances and rapidly develop severe symptoms that often leave them partially or even totally incapacitated.

Although progression of MS is unpredictable, several scoring systems have been developed through the years to measure its progress. The most common of these is the Kurtzke Disability Status Scale (DDS). Here, in abbreviated form, is how it works:

0— Normal neurological exam without any signs of disease present.
1— Slightly abnormal signs, but no symptoms.

2— Slight disability in a single body function.

3— Moderate disability in a single body function. Patient walks independently.

4— Severe disability in a single body function. Patient still can walk independently.

5— Severe disability, severely impaired walking. Patient is not able to work a full day.

6— Ambulatory aid such as a cane required for walking.

7— The patient is confined to a wheelchair, and can only walk several minutes a day.

8— The patient is fully confined to a wheelchair or bed, and cannot walk at all. The patient's arm movements remain intact.

9— Patient is fully confined to bed and has little or no use of limbs.

10— Death.

Know that the Kurtzke Disability Status Scale is an estimate, not a prediction, and that most MS patients will probably not experience most of the advanced stages listed in the higher scores.

Realize too that although the stages in the Kurtzke Scale are sequenced in order of increasing severity, individual experiences of MS will not necessarily conform to this chronology; that although persons may reach the fourth stage or fifth stage at one time or another they may then remit, returning to stages 1 or 2. To quote a passage from *The Parkinson's Disease Handbook*, which in this case is applicable to all medical staging systems as well: "None of the currently used means of evaluating [the disease] measure a patient's initiative, determination, spirit, or drive—all qualities which can transcend the patient's disability."*

Who will progress? Who will progress rapidly? Who will remit? Who will go into permanent remission?

The answer is simply not known. MS works according to

*A.S. Lieberman, G. Gopinathan, A. Neophytides, and M. Goldstein, *The Parkinson's Disease Handbook*. New York: American Parkinson's Disease Association (n.d.), p. 15.

mysterious laws of its own, and there are no absolute benchmarks to hang one's hat on. Middle-aged and young, male and female, strong and weak, fat and thin, black, white, yellow, brown—none of these factors seem to affect the rate of the disease's progression once a person develops it. For this reason multiple sclerosis has been called, somewhat tongue-in-cheek no doubt, a "democratic" disease.

One final point should be noted concerning the progressive and relapsing-progressive forms of MS. It is often claimed in medical literature that the course this disease takes during the first four or five years after its onset can be a predictive indication of how it will continue to reveal itself throughout a patient's lifetime.

Thus, if a person has a mild early attack that presents and remits with relative swiftness, and is then followed by only one or two small flareups in the next several years, this is a probable—*probable*—indication that the course of the condition will remain mild and manageable for the rest of that person's life. If severe symptoms show themselves from the beginning, especially in the functions of movement, gait, and coordination, and if these symptoms recur with increasing frequency and seriousness in the next several years, this may indicate that progression will be swift.

MS AND GEOGRAPHY

One of the most fascinating aspects of multiple sclerosis is its epidemiologic tendency to conform to predictable geographical patterns.

For example, MS is most frequently seen in the so-called "temperate zones" of the earth located between the 40-degree and 60-degree longitudinal bands, both north and south.

At the same time, the disease is practically unknown at the equator. Moreover, the farther north one moves, the greater the number of cases of MS that are reported.

This means that if you live at 10 degrees longitude, just above or below the equator, your chances of developing multiple sclerosis are less than if you live at 20 degrees longitude, above or below.

If you live at 20 degrees longitude your chances are less than if you live at 30 degrees, and so on up (or down) to the 40-to-60-degree danger areas of the temperate regions.

Several theories have been put forward to explain this peculiar relationship between MS and geographic habitat. One suggests that the high-incidence countries of the world are mostly situated in the temperate zones, where living conditions are sanitary and hygienic. Persons living in these countries, this line of reasoning holds, are not exposed as children to some unidentified X virus that may cause MS, and do not develop immunity. Children who live in poorer, less hygienic environments, on the other hand, are exposed to the theorized virus and thus may develop a natural form of resistance to it.

Perhaps. At the same time, however, industrialized countries located in the same temperate latitudes often show strikingly different frequency rates of MS, and consistent epidemiological patterns within adjacent regions are notoriously difficult to pinpoint.

For this reason some researchers claim that persons living in warmer climates have developed resistance to MS over the centuries and are genetically less susceptible to the virus, or to whatever the causes of the ailment may happen to be. While there is some tangible evidence to this effect, there is also contradictory evidence to show that MS is an environmentally acquired disorder, and that patterns of age and migration are essential variables in determining who will or will not get the disease.

Age and Migration

An anomaly closely related to the geographical enigma is the fact that children who grow up in warm or tropical locales, and who then emigrate to northern countries at around twelve years of age or younger, eventually tend to show more or less the same high susceptibility to MS as those who have lived in northern countries all their lives. But if individuals remain in a warm climate until their late teenage years, say age eighteen or nineteen, then move north, they remain as immune to the disease as they might had they lived in a warm environment their entire lives.

The same process works in reverse as well. Children twelve or younger who move from a northern climate to a warm southern environment are as immune to the disease as those who have lived there all their lives. But teenagers of seventeen, eighteen, or nineteen who move to the tropics from the north are as vulnerable to MS as persons who have lived in the cooler latitudes for forty years.

These demographic facts seem to lend strong credence to the theory that some type of contagious process takes place during childhood and puberty, and that environmental exposure to a specific MS-causing factor—probably a virus—vastly increases one's chances of getting the disease.

Sounds reasonable. The only problem is that as yet there is no conclusive proof that any kind of MS-producing virus actually exists.

Thus, like the fact that MS is a new disease, the geographical and migrational realities of MS at first make one think there are clear-cut clues here for determining a cause and perhaps even a cure. When closely analyzed, however, these facts end up producing nothing more than tantalizing hints, contradictions, and ambiguous dead ends.

Race, Nationality, Country

Black men and women are approximately half as likely to get MS as white. Some black races in Africa such as the Bantu never get the disease at all. Oddly enough, neither do the gypsies.

Also immune for reasons difficult to understand—they live almost exclusively in northern climates where prevalence is high—are the Eskimos. Another northern group, the Lapps of Finland, are similarly immune. Orientals tend to get the disease far less commonly than Caucasions. Countries with the highest rates of incidence are all predominantly wealthy, industrialized, and white. These include Scandinavia, Canada (especially the southern parts), England, Ireland, western Russia, New Zealand, Australia, and to a lesser extent the northern areas of the United States.

MS AND AGE OF ONSET

Persons who are destined to develop multiple sclerosis usually do so between the ages of fifteen and forty-five, though it is widely believed that the origins of the disease appear within the body sooner, most likely during puberty. The average age of onset for men is twenty-eight, for women twenty-five.

Older persons, say those over fifty, rarely get MS. If they do, chances are that they have been harboring the disease for many years, perhaps with a symptom flareup now and then that went ignored or misdiagnosed. By and large, MS is a young person's disease.

MS AND GENDER

Women are approximately two-thirds more likely to develop multiple sclerosis than men. In some areas of the world the balance is even more heavily biased in the direction of the female sex.

There are some who believe this statistic to be explainable by factors other than gender. Dr. Louis J. Rosner and Shelley Ross have the following interesting slant on the issue:

> Which survey should be accepted? Perhaps none. Taken on face value, they seem to indicate that MS has a definite preference for women, but other factors must be considered. At great risk of sounding sexist, it is our belief that women, in general, pay more attention to their health and see their doctors much more often than do men. So, although surveys show that more women than men contract MS, it is possible that the statistics are weighted in their favor simply because they make themselves more available for neurological assessments.*

---

*In *Multiple Sclerosis: New Hope and Practical Advice for People with MS and Their Families.* New York, Prentice-Hall Press, 1987, p. 10.

MS AND GENETIC INVOLVEMENT

Is multiple sclerosis directly inherited?

No, it is not. Yet there is a factor to be considered here that indicates some hereditary involvement: persons with family members who suffer from multiple sclerosis have a slightly increased *susceptibility*.

What, exactly, is the difference between genetic inheritance and susceptibility?

When a disease is hereditary it can potentially be transmitted from parent to child by means of a specific abnormal gene or set of genes. In some cases the probabilities of a person's developing such a genetically inherited disease can be statistically calculated. For example, a neurological ailment such as Huntington's chorea is clearly a genetic disorder; all offspring of a parent carrying its genes have a 50 percent chance of acquiring it by the time they are fifty years old. Genetic tests are even available that determine with 95 percent accuracy whether or not children of Huntington parents are carrying these abnormal genes.

Multiple sclerosis, on the other hand, also has a genetic component, but it tends to be a very small one. Roughly speaking, if there is MS in a person's family his or her chances of developing the disease are raised to a factor of around 1 in 50 to 100, as compared to the 1 in 1,000 figure for persons born with an MS-free family history.

The closer the blood relative the greater the risk. This means that if persons have cousins or uncles with MS their chances of acquiring it are a good deal less than if they have fathers or mothers with the disease. In the case of identical twins, if one of the twins has MS there is as much as a 70 percent chance that the other will get it too (in fraternal twins there is only about a 3 percent chance of this occurring). In 4 percent of families affected by multiple sclerosis, two or more close family members have the disease.

We have already seen that certain ethnic groups such as the Eskimos and Bantus rarely get MS, and this may be further indication that some type of hereditary factor is at work. There are other incriminating clues as well. One example is that the white blood cells of many persons with MS show a pattern of "human leukocyte antigens" (HLA) different from those of healthy persons. HLAs are believed to play a part in the human immune response, perhaps in fighting off infection. Since the patterns these antigens form themselves into are passed on by inheritance, and since persons with MS often show a certain HLA pattern in their cells, researchers are eagerly looking into the question of whether or not they represent a gene type or formation that makes their carriers more susceptible.

And yet, despite this and much other evidence, we also know that the environment plays a large part in the MS picture. It has even been suggested by some medical researchers that MS is less hereditary than statistics would have us believe, and that the actual reason persons with a family history of MS acquire it more frequently is that they are all exposed during childhood to some as yet unknown MS virus within the family household.

The fact of the matter is, however, that genetic susceptibility seems to be a very real phenomenon in the MS story, and is presently the subject of intensive scientific research. A likely theory is that MS susceptibility is genetically transmitted via several genes at once, or by a specific combination of genes, rather than through a single guilty gene alone; and that MS-carrying families pass this pattern on through the generations. As of 1992, a well-funded project sponsored by the National Multiple Sclerosis Society, known as "Genomic Search for Susceptibility Genes in Multiple Sclerosis," is investigating this possibility. Taking eighty or more families which appear to carry some kind of genetic code for MS, the research team is searching for genes and gene combinations that are responsible for susceptibility. Once this information is compiled, they then plan to determine what part each of these factors plays in the cause and development of multiple sclerosis.

CAUSES OF MULTIPLE SCLEROSIS

Perhaps no other neurological disease has generated as large a literature and as many etiological theories explaining its possible cause as MS. Over the years allergies, emotional liability, head traumas, pollution, thrombosis, hormonal imbalance, lack of essential fats in the diet, and many other explanations have been put forward, none of which stand up to the test of clinical examination. The theories that presently command the most respect and attention are:

1. Heredity
2. Autoimmune response
3. Virus
4. A combination of numbers 2 and 3 above.

We have already discussed heredity. It is clearly a significant variable, though probably less important in explaining the actual cause of central nervous system demyelination than the second, third, and fourth theories presented above. Let's have a look at each of these one at a time.

Autoimmune Response

The job of the human immune system is to rid the body of alien microscopic substances—viruses, allergens, bacteria, abnormal cells, and other potential troublemakers—by manufacturing antibodies and a type of white blood cell known as lymphocytes, which hunt down and destroy these invaders.

Located throughout the body in strategic areas such as the thymus gland, spleen, tonsils, adenoids, lymph nodes, and bone marrow, the immune system ordinarily performs its duties with miraculous efficiency. Take, for instance, the lymphocytes. There are approximately a trillion of these white blood cells in a healthy person's system at any given moment, and in a normal lifetime the immune system will produce a billion trillion more. Indeed, in the time it has taken you to read this page your body has already produced several million, each of which is unique, like snowflakes.

Although we have such powerful and prolific allies on our side it is an ironic fact of nature that occasionally, for reasons not entirely understood, the immunological system becomes confused and turns its formidable powers against its own host organism, causing a number of possible disturbances, including inflammation, toxicity, and destruction of healthy body tissue. A relatively long list of maladies, both common and uncommon, are set off by this process, technically known as a *hypersensitivity reaction*. Allergies are a relatively mild example. More serious are diabetes mellitus, Addison's disease, rheumatoid arthritis, rheumatic fever, and systemic lupus erythematosus.

At the present time many medical researchers believe that multiple sclerosis is also triggered by some variety of autoimmune process. Specifically, it is theorized that certain types of lymphocytes, known as T-cells, misread messages received from the myelin tissue, mistake it for an alien invader, attack it, and invite other immune cells to join them in the assault. This case of mistaken identity produces tissue damage to the myelin sheath, with consequent swelling and inflammation, and ultimately leads to the formation of sclerotic plaques.

Many studies have been conducted over the past few years to determine how well the autoimmune theory holds up under laboratory conditions, and the results are highly interesting. In one study, for example, rabbits were given a piece of rabbit nervous system mixed with an immune stimulator, usually a protein derived from the tuberculosis bacillus. Observation then showed that rabbits subjected to this test underwent an autoimmune reaction to these materials, becoming allergic to their own brains and developing patches of inflammation and demyelination very similar to the kind found in multiple sclerosis.

MS patients themselves, moreover, have shown evidence that their cellular immunity is different from that of persons without MS. Suppose that under laboratory conditions a doctor takes immune cells from an MS person and from a normal patient. The doctor then exposes these cells to a foreign substance, say a virus of some kind, such as mumps or measles, and measures the reaction of the cells in both control groups—how fast they attack the foreign substance and how fast they elaborate antibodies. Results have shown that basic differences in cell reaction exist between the two test groups, and that the cells of MS persons tend to produce an autoimmune type of response more often than those of persons without MS.

Does this imply that MS is caused by a virus? Yes, it does. But which one? And how?

The Virus Theory

Viruses are infectious agents considerably smaller in size than the smallest bacteria. They are responsible for producing a wide spectrum of ailments ranging from the common cold to warts, mumps, and AIDS.

When invading the human body, a virus's strategy of attack is to infiltrate larger host cells and once there to quickly replicate itself until a microscopic army of cloned viruses emerge, causing whatever ailment this particular organism is capable of producing.

To date, no one has been able to isolate or propagate a virus that can be positively identified as causing MS. Nonetheless, a suspicious trail has been picked up that points to the presence of *some* variety of viral infection and contamination.

Certain researchers, for example, believe that a virus may infiltrate the body and then trigger the type of autoimmune reaction described above. Others believe that a virus enters the body and attacks the immune system directly, confusing and disturbing it in such a way that it turns against itself. In several studies it has been demonstrated that approximately one-third of persons with MS report having suffered some type of viral infection immediately before the onset of their disease. When spinal taps are done on MS patients, moreover, one of the indicators of MS is a high antibody count in the fluid, a persuasive indicator that some kind of microorganism is being attacked by the immune system.

It is also known, as we have seen, that environmental factors play a large part in the development of multiple sclerosis. And it is believed by some medical professionals that in warm countries with low standards of living, children may be exposed to the theorized MS virus and develop an immunity to it. This would explain why people who live in tropical, less sanitary parts of the world almost never contract the disease. We know, moreover, that a similar process takes place with polio, and that people in poor countries who are exposed to the polio virus as children develop antibodies against it that protect them in high-exposure situations.

It has also been suggested by researchers that in certain northern countries where MS is rampant persons may be more likely to be born with a genetic susceptibility to the purported MS virus than those born in countries where the incidence is low. We know that among Scandinavians, who are especially prone to MS, the incidence of this disease remains relatively high among adults and small children alike, even when they emigrate to other countries.

What type of virus might be responsible for causing MS?

Various forms of influenza have been studied. So has herpes simplex and a retrovirus related to the AIDS virus known as HTLV−1. Some believe the culprit to be a form of rubeola or measles, though exhaustive research has failed to turn up anything conclusive. We know that measles is capable of producing another neurological disorder known as *sub-acute sclerosing panencephalitis*, a disease that produces dementia and inflammation in the brains of children, and that antibodies against the measles virus are found in the spinal fluid of three-quarters of MS patients. There are other indications implicating the measles virus as well, but none have yet provided decisive proof of any kind.

Interestingly enough, several decades ago a study was done based on a series of interviews with MS patients to determine the constants in their lifestyles. Among the many pieces of information revealed was that MS patients seem more likely than non-MS patients to have owned a small dog sometime in their past.

This fact is not as trivial as it seems, as the virus which produces canine distemper has come on the firing line as a possible producer of MS. It has been reported in *Neurology* (April 1985), for instance, that in the Orkney Islands off Scotland, where MS rates are among the highest in the world, the incidence of MS rose during the Second World War when soldiers brought their dogs with them to the islands, then dropped off dramatically several decades later when the canine population, along with the incidence of distemper, declined.

Like so many promising viral theories, however, no one has yet produced clinical proof that distemper—or any other virus-caused disease—is definitely linked to MS. At the same time the evidence for viral involvement is too strong to disregard. Many doctors now believe that the cause of the disease may ultimately prove to involve both a virus *and* an autoimmune response.

Combined Autoimmunity and Virus

Let's take one possible scenario. At the age of thirteen, a teenage girl is exposed to a particular virus. She suffers a sore throat and fever perhaps, and other symptoms of the flu. Then she gets better.

In the process of fighting off this ailment her immune system develops antibodies and immune cells that are specifically designed and programmed to rid the body of this particular virus. Owing to some peculiarity within the targeted virus, however, and perhaps to some inherited tendency within the girl's immune system, the virus looks a good deal like the myelin lining in the girl's nervous system. In the future, therefore, when these immune cells happen to come across nerve tissue in the myelin sheath, the information bank that drives them mistakes the tissue for the virus, and the cells attack it. Inflammation and demyelination result; MS begins.

This is one possible scenario among many involving a virus and autoimmune reaction. Another is that a certain virus attacks the immune system and disorients it in such a way that the immune system becomes inactive when a second virus, the one actually responsible for causing MS, enters the system. It is also possible that several viruses attacking in concert are the guilty parties. At the present time there is little evidence to show that a single virus acting directly on its own in the way that, say, a flu virus does, can produce the disease. Whatever the ultimate etiology of MS happens to be, however, it most likely involves a complex interaction that has to be studied many years before it is completely understood.

There are several other variations on this interesting theme that are currently being investigated. Scientists are, in fact, pursuing this line of study with great intensity and optimism today, and no doubt we shall learn a great deal more about the inner chemistry responsible for MS in the next few years.

2

MS—Is It or Isn't It?

Let's suppose that you have recently developed a case of blurred vision. Or that one of your legs, normally a pillar of steadiness, becomes inexplicably weak at moments during the day. Perhaps you feel the urge to urinate more often than before. Or you have numbness in your legs.

Are you suffering from MS?

Certainly all these symptoms are possible signs of the disease. But does having one or even several of them warrant sounding the alarm?

Most likely not. Because any of these symptoms may be caused by dozens of other physical problems as well. For this reason, multiple sclerosis is a rather difficult disease to diagnose, especially in its early stages.

The disease's development is unpredictable, and the types of symptoms it produces are occasionally unusual and difficult to track to their source. Even when a person displays several MS-like symptoms at once, this by no means offers conclusive proof of a diagnosis. Only after ruling out a list of other possible causes *plus* several MS look-alike disorders, and then finding clinical evidence for the disease itself can a medical decision be reached.

One is therefore cautioned against jumping to conclusions. "You don't got it till you got it," as the old-time physicians used to say. Take the case of Irene P.

A woman in her middle twenties, Irene has always been athletic, especially in her college years when she starred on her school's equestrian team (and where she came close to winning a national championship). Since that time she has remained physically active, faithfully following a daily regime of aerobics, and running whenever she has time.

One day, as Irene was jogging near her home, she suddenly, and quite uncharacteristically, lost her balance and fell to the ground.

Nothing like this had ever happened before. Several days later, sure enough, the same thing occurred, the same unexplained loss of balance and buckling at the knees. It was frightening.

Now Irene happened to have several cases of MS in her family, and she was well versed in the facts concerning its onset. Wasn't sudden loss of balance a major symptom—especially when it tended to happen at odd, unexpected times for no apparent reason?

When these episodes continued she quickly became convinced that she was falling victim to MS, just like her grandfather and uncle. Several sleepness nights followed.

But was she? In fact, she was not. Her loss of balance, it turned out, was caused by a reaction to an allergy medication she was taking. As soon as she learned this fact she stopped taking the drug, and the balance loss and falling never occurred again.

The moral is an important one. As trained clinicians will invariably agree, MS is a sickness in which a little knowledge can be a particularly dangerous thing. Many persons learn a few facts about the disease, hear a few horror stories from friends, watch a few scare shows on TV, and before long every tingling of the toes or slip on the ice becomes cause for alarm. Such people are thoroughly convinced that they have MS. But usually they don't. Usually their problems can be traced to a more common cause.

WHEN SHOULD I BE WORRIED?

The question then arises: When, in fact, does a person have real cause for suspecting MS involvement? When is it time to get serious about one's symptoms and schedule a visit to the family physician, or even to a neurologist?

The following model situations present a general answer to this important question. Each of these models profiles an instance in which a consultation with a physician is appropriate. Each is a possible cause for concern. Again, restraint must be added to the picture; and remember that it is counterproductive to make writ-in-stone assumptions about the state of your health until a doctor has conducted an exam.

With these cautions remembered, take note of the following:

1. A person experiences several of the most common MS symptoms in a relatively short period of time. A sampling of these symptoms may include visual disturbances (such as blurred vision, inability to see directly from the center of the eye, double vision), bladder difficulties (frequent urination, inability to fully void the bladder, loss of bladder control), gait disorders, numbness or tingling in the extremities or other parts of the body, and sudden coordination loss. Be concerned if several of these complaints occur at the same time, or if one of them is increasingly persistent.

2. A person experiences a single MS-like symptom such as any of the above, and this symptom continues for several weeks or months. Bladder or urinary trouble, for example, is a common complaint in many people's lives at one time or another, and is usually nothing to be alarmed about. But if a bladder problem makes a person uncomfortable for several weeks in a row, and if the condition becomes increasingly serious, a trip to the doctor is advised. At worst, the doctor will tell you what it is—or isn't—and treat the condition accordingly.

3. If either of the above scenarios does occur, even to a minor degree, *and* you (1) are between the ages of fifteen and forty-five; (2) were born and brought up in a northern or temperate climate;

(3) have a family history of MS, why not get it checked? The example of Irene, the woman with the family history of MS given above, was presented not to criticize her concern, only to warn against premature alarm.

WHAT ARE THE MOST COMMON SYMPTOMS OF MS?

Keeping the above facts in mind, let's take a more detailed look at some typical symptoms that may occur with MS.

The first thing to realize is that MS takes a wide variety of forms. These include mental and emotional disturbances as well as physical. Almost any symptom characteristic of a central nervous system disorder can be a symptom of MS as well.

Be aware too that when symptoms first show themselves they tend to last for several weeks or longer before subsiding. One to three months is the average time it takes them to run their full course.

After the first attack these symptoms may never come back, and the person may go on to live life in a state of permanent remission. Or the symptoms may return. This could happen in a month, or a year, or a decade, or several decades. There is no way of being sure.

Even when persons have symptoms, moreover, most continue to lead active, participating lives, and many learn to deal with their handicaps in an impressively efficient and courageous manner. To reiterate what was said in Chapter 1: approximately 20 percent of patients will experience a single attack and never be bothered again. Ten percent will experience symptoms that become permanent and quickly progress, sometimes to the point of incapacitation. The remaining 70 percent will have symptoms that appear, disappear, than reappear again at varying intervals of time and degrees of severity.

What physical complications might a patient expect to encounter? The following are the most frequent symptoms reported by persons with MS.

1. Visual disorders— One of the most frequent early signs of MS is eye trouble. Patients may experience a blurring of vision, usually in one eye. Seen objects appear murky, as if one were looking at the world through water; or a kind of opaque blind spot known as a *cecocentral scotoma* forms in the center of the field of vision, sometimes spreading slowly outward and cutting off a person's straight-ahead view. Double vision is also a possibility.

Leslie H., a newly diagnosed MS patient, tells of her first encounter with a vision problem:

> I was driving to work. It was still dark in winter. Normally, I wear glasses while driving, though my eyes are mostly fine. I went over the railroad tracks and approached the stoplight in the center of town when all of a sudden the red light lost its color and became pale, blurry. Fuzzy. I rubbed my eyes and took off my glasses, but it continued. It must have gone on about a minute. Then everything went back to normal. A few days later the same thing happened to me while I was watching TV.

As in Leslie's case, attacks of visual impairment tend to be transient, sometimes lasting only minutes or even seconds. Such episodes are caused by inflammation around the optic nerve, a condition known as *optic neuritis*, which is produced by the demyelinating lesions that form on its sensitive tissue. When this lesion heals, as it tends to do, normal sight returns, sometimes completely, sometimes with vision slightly impaired or with small blind spots in the field of focus. Even when a person becomes partially or totally blind, however, as occasionally happens, this condition almost always passes; permanent blindness among MS patients is a rarity.

Note also that when optic neuritis does take place, even when unaccompanied by other symptoms, its presence can be a warning sign of problems to come. Such attacks tend to return, often in the company of other symptoms this time, though it may take years or even decades before this happens.

On the other hand, there are many people who walk around all their lives with undiagnosed optic neuritis; and there are people who suffer only a single attack. Statistically speaking, in approximately one-half of all cases an episode of optic neuritis will be followed by symptoms of MS within the next days, months, or years to come.

When sight problems persist, ophthalmic assistance plus corticosteroid medications, prescription glasses, eye patches, stress reduction, and simple rest may all help. Other eye symptoms characteristic of MS include defective color vision, nystagmus (a condition in which the eye makes jerky, involuntary oscillating movements), weakness of night vision, and an oversensitivity to light. All these conditions can be exacerbated by tension, eye strain, and fatigue.

2. Speech abnormalities— We talk and make sounds with our lips, throat, palate, vocal cords, and tongue. Key control centers for these parts are located in the brain stem and cerebellum, areas frequently affected by MS. It is thus not unusual for an MS patient to talk in a hesitant, slurred, and/or arrhythmic voice.

In many persons, especially those in the early stages of the disease, this defect can be slight, so slight that the patient is unaware of its existence. To complicate matters, conscious and unconscious compensations may be devised to disguise it. To the outside world these defects thus sound like a simple slowness of articulation, not an unusual trait in healthy people. The voice may have a slight slur to it or even a kind of offbeat, sometimes charmingly eccentric rhythm.

Laymen fail to identify these oddities as speech defects per se. But a trained clinician, especially if he or she already suspects MS, will be listening for them throughout the neurological examination. In many cases speech problems can be helped by a speech therapist, especially when the difficulty lies in slurring and arrhythmical speech, symptoms known medically as *dysarthria*.

More problematic, and fortunately a good deal less common, are swallowing disorders. When these occur patients must force their swallowing muscles to work, often with a good deal of struggle. While eating they may choke, even on soft foods—especially on soft foods—or get food lodged at the back of their throats. These difficulties occur because the complex set of muscles involved in the swallowing mechanism stop working in proper coordination during the swallowing process. Again, speech therapists can be of help in advising patients how to avoid swallowing problems and in suggesting shortcuts to improvement.

3. Movement, coordination, and balance problems— Problems with movement and coordination are frequent in MS, especially in the limbs, and particularly in the legs. As many persons have discovered, such symptoms are often the first to be noted when MS strikes.

Patients may discover, for instance, that movements they have always performed in an automatic way suddenly go awry. One female patient talked of walking across her kitchen holding a pie plate when, for no apparent reason, the plate slipped from her hands. Another, a worker at a glass factory who spends many hours of the day seated, developed a sudden clumsiness and inability to coordinate her legs when she got in and out of her chair. Occasionally she fell. A third woman had trouble gripping her pen after several minutes of writing.

Anita M., a woman in her early thirties, speaks of her first experience with coordination difficulties:

> My leg started acting funny. It felt as if one leg was longer than the other. And it sometimes got numb. It was like a jellyfish inside, not numb really, but like if you were sticking it with a needle. In the mornings it felt like it was heavy, like the circulation was not good. This was in one leg only, in my right leg. The left never has bothered me. At first it didn't cause me any problems walking. I could make it look straight. Then everybody started telling me I was walking stupid. So I'd swing it from my hip to make it look straight. After a while it got so it hurt my hip. I got so I walked slow and would even stagger. My boyfriend would tell me not to "walk funny." It makes my lower back sore. I get a lot of muscle spasms. Sometimes my leg will sort of jump. It's hard to explain.

As in Anita's case, gait problems are a common early sign of MS, and ambulation disabilities are often part of a patient's overall symptom picture. A person may have a leg go out from under him or her for no traceable reason. He or she may be riding a bicycle and for several minutes find it impossible to coordinate the pedaling motions. The person may be climbing stairs and suddenly be unable to take the next step. The difficulty can manifest as a slight limp, as in Anita's case, a dragging, shuffling weakness, or in-turning of the foot. In still other cases, as a result of damage to cerebellar connections in the brain, lurching and wobbliness will occur, and a cane may temporarily become necessary to help the person remain steady. This type of motor incoordination and the jerky, shaking movements that accompany it is medically known as *ataxia*, a condition that can occur in the upper extremities as well, producing an inability to orchestrate arm movements and a tendency to "overshoot" when reaching for objects. At times, moreover, the particularly clumsy, staggering gait characteristic of ataxia makes a patient appear drunk or drugged. Indeed, one of the psychological problems that people afflicted with gait disorders must cope with is the fear that others will look on them as inebriated rather than walking-impaired.

In a small number of cases a gait condition can progress to the point where a person is incapacitated and even wheelchair-bound. Again, though, even the most serious episodes of motor disturbance sometimes go into remission. When this occurs most, if not all, of a person's coordination returns.

4. Numbness and tingling— Numbness and tingling are another set of symptoms typical of MS. A patch of skin on the arm may feel dead to the touch or produce a pins-and-needles feeling, a condition known as *paresthesia*. Surface sensations of burning, cold, or sharp, shooting pains are sometimes experienced. Skin areas can become unusually sensitive to the touch, producing discomfort, even under light pressure, a response medically known as *dysesthesia*.

We are all familiar with one or more of these sensations, especially pins-and-needles. The feeling is similar to when a foot falls asleep, or when we are recuperating from a case of frostbite, or when a wound is healing. There are a number of variations. With MS, however, these symptoms appear out of the blue, then recur with annoying regularity without any apparent reason. Is this cause for alarm? The rule of thumb is: If minor numbness, skin surface pain, or tingling comes and goes without other MS-like symptoms accompanying it, there is probably nothing to worry about, especially when the condition moves to different locations and disappears quickly. If these sensations arrive in the company of one or more of the MS symptoms mentioned above and then persist, keep a close watch on their development, especially if they are located in the feet, legs, and trunk areas.

The notion that a symptom occurs "out of the blue," however, bears examination. Occasionally, for example, a patient will complain of sudden numbness, or sudden symptoms of any kind, and then, when the medical history is taken, it is revealed that he or she experienced attacks of this type in the past and promptly forgot them. This may be due partly to the fact that memory is affected in some MS patients, partly to the understandable fact that when a symptom goes away on its own we stop thinking about it.

In one case a woman complained of numbness in her feet and left hand. After taking her history it became evident that she had experienced similar symptoms years before and had been having weakness in an intermittent fashion for some time without realizing it. Making allowances for her memory, which in this case was poor, it was clear that she had overlooked these symptoms in the past and simply put them out of her head. Now, seventeen years after the first signs of the disease showed themselves, she was in a doctor's office receiving a diagnosis of MS.

Note this point also. When all is said and done, numbness and tingling are two of the *least* reliable indicators of MS. This is true for a number of reasons but mainly because such complaints are indicative of dozens of other problems as well, ranging from sciatica and a tight belt, to anemia and vitamin B (thiamin) deficiency, to peripheral vascular disease, diabetes, and toothache. Or to nothing in particular that any physician can identify.

A good example of a disorder that produces MS-like skin sensation is *carpal tunnel syndrome*. Here the median nerve of the arm gets uncomfortably squeezed and pinched in a tunnel of tendons as it passes through the wrist, ultimately causing the hand

and/or the arm to turn numb. Persons who use their hands a great deal—factory employees, typists, computer operators, workers who cut with scissors many hours a day—are all prone to carpal tunnel. Most of them live with this condition for years without thinking much about it. A few become alarmed and pay a visit to the doctor's office, afraid that they may have MS. They don't.

Note on numbness: It has been stated by many patients that when numbness and tingling are given too much attention—when one obsesses over the problem—it tends to get worse. Since numbness is a relatively harmless condition that causes little pain and no damage, patients are advised to ignore it as best they can and accept it as a niggling but relatively minor annoyance. The more power it is given the more aggravating it becomes. There is presently no medication that can be taken to relieve numbness.

---

5. Altered mental condition— There has always been confusion over the topic of MS and mental condition. On the one hand, it was believed for many years that MS did not affect cognitive abilities, and that whatever mental slips occurred among patients were due to secondary causes such as depression. At the same time, before a good deal was known about the disease, doctors and nurses who dealt with MS became collectively vexed over the fact that MS patients seemed inconsistent and irrational in their reporting of symptoms, complaining this month of eye problems, the next of walking disorders, the third of incontinence, with new and seemingly unrelated disorders turning up on a regular basis. Many medical professionals dismissed this series of seemingly unrelated and illogical complaints as evidence that MS persons in general were either cranks or slightly daft. Today we know that such shifting symptomology is a fundamental part of the disease.

It is now understood that MS can, in fact, exert a negative influence on cognitive capacity, though usually to a limited degree. Since the mind with its seemingly limitless array of mental functions is controlled by the central nervous system, a sclerosis forming in the brain may produce alterations in the higher mental functions, such as thought, concentration, memory, and mood. Even the emotions are not immune, being under the command of the brain as well.

When such changes occur, a variety of responses are possible. People may find they cannot concentrate as well as before. They may need to pace themselves while performing difficult thought tasks such as reading a textbook or solving a math problem. Memory can be affected, as can judgment. Mood swings are not unusual, though other possible explanations exist for such behavior, including depression or the side effects of medication. Occasionally, to the chagrin of caregivers, advanced patients will become increasingly insensitive to the world around them, withdrawing or losing interest in matters of daily living; or worse perhaps, becoming heedless of social norms and behaving in ways that are embarrassing for everyone, it seems, but the patient.

In most cases, however, the mental deficits that do develop are slight and are often undetectable to anyone but patients and their families. MS sufferers, for example, may notice a certain slowness in their mental reaction time, and in their method of self-expression, a kind of gentle vagueness that others read as mood, fatigue, or simply as an element of the person's personality. In rare cases, a psychosis such as schizophrenia or manic-depression can also appear or become exacerbated, but usually only if a person has been prone to such problems before the onset of their MS.

Many MS patients, it should also be said, experience no negative mental symptoms of any kind. As with all things in this disease, the verdict is never in till it's in. Gina B., a woman of twenty-three, has been diagnosed with a case of MS for several years. She speaks on the subject of her mental symptoms:

I have trouble, I guess you'd say, remembering short-term kinds of stuff now. Names, phone numbers. I used to be pretty good at it. My long-term memory is fine though. I compensate by putting things I know I'll need in their right order. Like, I have a stack of coasters in my apartment and I always keep my keys on top of them now. I put things in reach in my closet to keep tabs on where they are. That kind of thing. I also find that sometimes my better judgment is affected. In social matters. With friends. In arguments. I sometimes do or say things I regret later. This is true when I'm tired, mostly.

Megan R., also twenty-three years old, has experienced a number of concentration problems since she first showed signs of MS at age eighteen.

A definite problem for me is my concentration. I'll start talking about the things I want to do and then I'll lose track of them real easy. I study for a while at school. I used to sit reading for three or four hours at a time. Now I put my work down when my concentration starts to fuzz, usually within twenty minutes or so. I get up and go do something else for a while, then I come back to it. This helps to break my studying into intervals. I can concentrate fine in short bursts. I'm just not so great at the long haul.

Technically speaking, depression can also be a symptom of MS, especially when it appears *before* the diagnosis has been made, and particularly when it accompanies other MS-like complaints.

But here one stands on tentative ground. The experience of discovering that one has MS can plummet a person into the doldrums, producing episodes of anxiety, nerves, and general feelings of despair. This person then assumes that his or her distress is caused by the disease when in fact it is simply a quite understandable reaction to the diagnosis.

In other instances persons fall into depression during chemotherapy, only to learn that it is medicine that is getting them down, not the disease. The waters here get murky. In many cases, probably a majority, depression is a psychological reaction to the disease of MS, not a symptom produced by it. In later sections we will discuss this issue, especially in regard to its effects on patients' mental attitudes and on their level of day-to-day emotional functioning.

6. Spasticity— A primary cause of motor disability, especially in the legs and postural muscles, is a muscle condition known as *spasticity*. Spasticity occurs when the groups of muscles that ordinarily tighten and relax to produce normal ambulation lose their capacity to work together properly, producing an increase in tone (tone is a muscle's ability to resist an applied external force), with stiffness and tightening in the affected limb.

This change in muscle tone is of a very specific kind for the MS patient. In other neurological diseases such as Parkinson's disease, tone alterations produce a steady rigidity of the limb. In MS, however, increase in tone reveals itself as a firm resistance when the limb is first raised, then a sudden release and relaxation. For example, if a doctor quickly pulls up under an MS patient's knee, the leg will come up hard and straight, then after a moment go weak and soft. Though MS is not the only disease that causes spasticity, its presence can be an important diagnostic indication.

When spasticity occurs a person will discover that a great deal more effort must be expended in walking and getting around than before, with fewer results to show for it. A person's leg will tend to lock up, for instance; or it may give way entirely at times. One tends to limp, to drag the leg much in the way Anita has described above. Walking may appear jiggly or shaky, a typical indication, which at times is also the only visible clue that spasticity is present. Sometimes charley horse–like spasms occur, putting the limbs into painful contractions. In the arms it may manifest as a lack of coordination in the hands and fingers. Fortunately, there are medication and physical-therapy techniques to help alleviate this condition in many patients. Both will be discussed in later chapters.

A related but quite different condition, known as *hypotonia*, can also bother patients at times. Hypotonia occurs when the muscle tone of a limb becomes entirely absent and the limb responds to manipulation much in the manner of a rag doll, with little or no resistance at all. On the whole, hypotonia is a good deal less common in MS persons than spasticity.

7. Tremor— In a number of neurological ailments a patient will have a tremor that vibrates at a relatively steady rate. The characteristic tremor of Parkinson's disease, for instance, oscillates at four to seven cycles a second; for a benign essential tremor the rate is around fifteen to twenty cycles per second. With MS the oscillation and its degree of intensity are less consistent and tend to vary widely from person to person. In some patients the movement is a barely discernible few cycles a second. In others it is a good deal faster and more noticeable.

Like most other neurological ailments, the timing of an MS tremor's arrival is predictable only in its unpredictability: it can come and go at any moment. Like other neurological ailments too, it may locate itself in many different parts of the body, including the hands, arms, feet, legs, trunk, and chin. Sometimes it appears in disguised form in a person's voice. Finally, like other ailments with a neurological basis, MS tremor is made worse when a person becomes excited, emotional, tense, or fatigued.

Over the years several rehabilitative strategies have been developed to control the shaking that occasionally afflicts patients. In a later chapter we will describe them in detail.

8. Weakness and fatigue— Patients will frequently complain to examining physicians that their legs are not lifting properly, that their fingers are clumsy and out of sync with one another, that their arms feel "heavy" all the time.

In fact, it is not so much lack of coordination that is causing this sensation but an overall weakness of the body parts.

This weakness presents patients with the illusion that the muscles in an arm or leg have "gone gushy on them," as one person put it. In reality, their muscular systems are working fine; it is the nerve pathways that have been disturbed. The result is a decrease in capacity to lift, pull, carry, grip, and push, depending on the motor function affected.

From the standpoint of the physician, these symptoms can often be a puzzlement and it may be difficult to know exactly which mechanism is at work—weakness, incoordination, or a combination of both. For the patient, it is all the same, however: a part of their body has become feeble, unresponsive, slow, and the going is rough.

Fatigue, on the other hand, exerts a more global weakening

effect over a person's entire body. Patients feel bone-tired for no particular reason. Their energy reserve is low at times of the day when they are normally most active. "It's as if God suddenly pulled my plug," one female patient said. Another described it as "like turning all of a sudden into rubber." Some persons become overwhelmed with an almost irresistible desire to lie down and sleep. Others need to make frequent stops when working or walking, or to take a series of planned rests during the day.

When fatigue does occur as part of MS, which is almost always the case, it is necessary for patients to avoid overdoing, even when exercising and undergoing physical therapy, and to develop methods for setting sensible limits on all their exertions. In other parts of this book we will discuss ways in which patients can learn to pace themselves and maximize their energy levels.

9. Bladder and bowel disorders— The bladder is a hollow sac located in the groin; its function is to serve as a kind of reservoir for holding urine before the command from the brain arrives to release it.

Composed mainly of muscle tissue plus a lining known as the urinary epithelium, the bladder can comfortably retain about a pint of fluid before it begins to reach overload. At the bottom of this sac a circular muscle known as the sphincter is situated, which in turn is connected to a long tube, the urethra, that transports urine down to the penis or vagina for excretion.

When the bladder fills and is stretched to the point of needing to empty itself, it sends "full" nerve messages to the spinal cord and brain, which in turn send signals back telling the sphincter to relax and the muscles of the bladder to contract and push the urine down and out. Successful urination is based on these two parts of the bladder system, the muscle wall and sphincter muscle, working in perfect coordination.

A relatively common early symptom of MS is a frequent and sometimes constant need to urinate. Most of us are capable of going an entire morning without acting on this urge more than, say, once or twice. With MS, however, the motor-control system that operates the bladder becomes defective owing to demyelinating plaques situated on the pathways from the brain to the bladder and back again. The bladder thus tends to become small and "spastic," and when given the neural message to eliminate it fails to perform on cue.

A variation on this theme occurs when the bladder sends voiding signals to the brain, and the brain, because of damage done to the myelin sheath, sends disturbed or faulty release signals back. The result is that the sphincter does not work in proper sync with the muscles of the bladder wall and fails to open and close as it should. Or conversely, the sphincter opens and remains open, while the bladder wall fails to push the urine out in a systematic way. In the first case, the urine builds up for long periods of time, the bladder expands beyond its retention capacity, and the urine leaks out involuntarily, causing wetness and embarrassment. In the second, constant, uncontrolled dribbling occurs.

When persons suffering from bladder problems finally do urinate, they may experience the uncomfortable sensation that their urine has not been thoroughly voided. A residual buildup, known as *retention,* remains and can pester a person throughout the day. In advanced stages, control over bladder function is lost entirely and incontinence results. In such cases temporary or even permanent catheterization may be required.

Because of inconsistent or incomplete voiding patterns, MS patients with bladder disorders often become prone to recurring urinary tract infections. These are due to the residual urine volume that remains stored in the bladder and acts there as a kind of culturing medium for infectious bacteria. Fortunately, medications and preventive measures can usually keep this problem in check.

Bladder dysfunction in MS is generally referred to as *neurogenic bladder.* There are several possible problems that can result from this condition, with many variations on the theme.

The first is storage dysfunction, whereby the bladder becomes incapable of holding even small amounts of urine. A person afflicted in this way feels a constant desire to urinate—urgency—and this sensation is produced, in turn, by involuntary muscle contractions of the shrunken bladder. The result is frequency, leaking, and sometimes complete loss of control over the urinary functions.

The second problem is voiding dysfunction where the sphincter and the muscles of the bladder wall fail to work in proper coordination. Here the sphincter tightens instead of relaxing when it is time to urinate, thus interfering and working against the bladder muscle's pushing motions. Or it may happen the other way around, in which case the sphincter opens but the bladder muscles fail to push. A certain amount of urine may then be excreted or dribbled out, but usually very little, and persons continue to feel the urge no matter how many times they void.

Voiding dysfunction can also produce *hesitancy,* an inability to urinate at will, whereby patients find themselves straining at the toilet for many minutes with only an insignificant amount of urination to show for it. Since the bladder is incapable of emptying itself properly when afflicted in this way, patients experience a runover effect, in which the urine comes out on its own, leaking and dribbling.

Though we will deal with treatment strategies for bladder disorders in a later chapter, it can be said here that persons suffering from residual retention can sometimes mitigate this problem *by sitting down to urinate*—this is important for men as well as women—then applying firm downward pressure to the abdomen with the palms, and massaging this area with firm, circular, downward motions, as if literally pressing out the urine. Also helpful is tightening the muscles in the bladder and urogenital areas, and literally "squeezing" out the excess. An anecdotal tip comes from a patient:

> In the beginning of my illness I often had a constant need to go number one. It drove me crazy. Every five minutes to the toilet. People thought I was crazy. I was able to hold my trips down thanks to a couple of tips I got from my mother. She told me to massage my lower stomach when I had that feeling, to take deep breaths, and to concentrate on relaxing the lower part of my body. I would do this while lying in bed sometimes and it helped, especially when I turned on my left side. It offered a little temporary relief in between those frantic dashes to the john. She also

told me to get rid of the extra urine that won't come out right away by standing up and sitting down a couple of times while I'm on the toilet, and then trying to pass my urine again. I don't know why this helps. It feels like a fresh start every time I stand up and sit down again.

Another potential bladder problem occurs when a combination of retention and voiding dysfunction gang up on the urinary function. Here the bladder is excessively active and at the same time the sphincter muscle behaves erratically and unpredictably. This combination produces hesitancy, urgency, incomplete voiding, burning bladder, and a condition of nighttime frequency known as *nocturia*.

A further potential source of eliminative trouble for MS sufferers is bowel disorder, which tends to affect relatively large numbers of patients. This condition, mainly constipation, is not typically produced by MS itself, though in some cases demyelination along the central nervous system will interfere with proper nerve transmission to the bowels, slowing the transit time of the feces through the digestive tract. More frequently, constipation is a response to nonpathological factors such as lack of adequate movement and exercise, side effects of medication, improper diet, low intake of liquids, and depression. In a later section we will profile accessible remedies that can be used to control constipation and reestablish regularity.

10. Sexual changes— MS can affect a patient sexually in two distinct ways, either directly through impairment of the nerve pathways that service and control the sexual functions, or in secondary ways through impairment of bladder function, spasticity, lack of energy, and depression.

Men who are sexually afflicted by MS most often complain of impaired ejaculation, decrease of sensation in the pleasure centers, and impotence. Women speak of a reduction in sensation in the vagina, feelings of stiffness and awkwardness during lovemaking, vaginal dryness, lack of ability to reach orgasm, and a general decrease in the sexual drive.

Despite such serious-sounding complaints, many patients

make satisfying and sometimes amazing adaptations to their deficits in this area. The subject of sexuality and MS is a complex one, and there are steps that can be taken to help. These and related matters will be discussed in a later chapter.

WHAT ABOUT PAIN?

Does it hurt to have MS?

Certainly it is a daunting experience to undergo urinary incontinence or impaired walking or confinement to a wheelchair. But can a newly diagnosed person also expect to be plagued by inordinate amounts of pain in the months and years that lie ahead?

Broadly speaking, most MS symptoms produce some degree of discomfort, but generally do not cause inordinate suffering. It has been estimated, for example, that approximately two-thirds of persons with multiple sclerosis are free of physical distress most if not all the time, and that their most frequent concerns, such as urinary problems and spasticity, are typified by feelings of discomfort rather than acute pain.

This, of course, leaves one-third of the MS population who may, in fact, experience some type of acute or chronic pain.

Of these, intense facial pain, known as *trigeminal neuralgia,* is probably the most disturbing and intense. Typified by sudden, lancinating jabs of pain on one side of the face (rarely, if ever, on both), facial neuralgia is caused by nerve disturbances along the pathway of the fifth cranial nerve, the sensory fibers of which run through the lower jaw, cheek, and lip.

The areas affected by this condition most commonly include the jaw, cheekbones, eye socket, forehead, and mouth. Frequently it is triggered by animated physical activity, especially activities that involve facial movement or facial exposure to the elements: chewing, talking excitedly, singing, puffing on a cigarette, sudden laughter, or a cold draft on the face. Several medicines exist that help reduce the pain of this disorder and keep it under control.

Another cause of facial pain, known as optic neuritis, usually occurs in one eye only, and often affects persons who are already undergoing MS-related vision problems. Triggering intense, hot pains from the optic nerve up to and behind the eyeball, episodes of optic neuritis tend to be transient, coming and going over a period of several weeks, then diminishing. Occasionally, attacks can lead to a slight though permanent reduction of function in the fine focusing mechanisms of the eye.

In some people paresthesia and dysesthesia are also problems. These isolated tender patches of irritation appear on different parts of the body, especially the lower parts, where they produce a burning or tingling sensation when touched. For most people they are simply a nuisance. For a few they produce genuine distress when pressed or rubbed. Even a shirt sleeve or a collar tab touching the problem area will produce discomfort.

Seizures are another difficult but relatively uncommon result of MS. Several varieties exist. Persons can experience an abrupt stiffening or paralysis on one side of the body. Or they may undergo a sudden paroxysm that in some ways resembles epilepsy. Such attacks usually last less than a minute and sometimes only for seconds. Tending to come in clusters, then subsiding, they affect a minuscule percent of the MS population and are usually not cause for concern.

Note too, as a kind of aside, that patients may suffer from several of the pain symptoms mentioned above and still show no clear signs of MS. One woman, for example, complained of facial neuralgia and seizures. She had originally been evaluated by a neurosurgeon who noted certain suspicious cerebellar symptoms and diagnosed a possible malignant tumor. A CAT scan was ordered and it showed that the side of her brain stem was indeed swollen. So the doctor opened up the woman's brain; and there, instead of a tumor, he saw only a red, swollen, angry bulge on her brain stem, clear indication that the real problem was not a tumor at all but multiple sclerosis.

Finally, it should be mentioned that pain can be triggered by complications secondary to the disease and not from the MS lesions directly. Persons with walking problems may develop secondary back pains or hip pains. Pinched nerves in the lower back are common. Persons who are immobilized by the disease suffer muscle spasms, contractures, circulatory ailments, and joint diseases such as arthritis. Eye pain may result from the intense squinting and strain caused by primary visual disturbances. Urinary infections result from chronic problems in the bladder. Pressure sores—decubiti—sometimes afflict those confined to a bed or wheelchair. Depression or anxiety can be brought on by the realization that one is suffering from a chronic neurological disease that is not going to go away.

In all, it is certainly no fun having MS, and in many cases heroic adjustments must be made to its discomforts. At the same time, among the various neurological diseases that afflict the human race, MS ranks among the *least likely* to inflict extreme physical pain. And this is a mark that can go on the plus side of the column when—and if—a diagnosis of MS is received.

3

Seeking a Diagnosis

A neurological diagnosis of MS is based on a number of variables that must come together in such a way that 1) the evidence pointing toward MS is present; 2) the evidence pointing away from it is eliminated.

Such a procedure takes time, sometimes more time than a patient may wish, and in certain cases a conclusive diagnosis will be impossible to reach on the first or second visit.

A diagnosis for MS, understand, is never an absolute certainty. After exhaustive tests, physical and mental neurological exams, lab work, plus careful consideration of all presented symptomology, a doctor may conclude that an examinee is suffering from MS; and chances are excellent that the diagnosis is accurate. At the same time, *no single definitive test for multiple sclerosis exists at the present time.* The only foolproof diagnostic method medicine possesses is an autopsy of a suspected MS patient's brain after death.

A clinical diagnosis of MS is therefore based both on the evidence presented by the patient, and on *a diagnosis of exclusion;* which means, in turn, that a doctor can assume a patient has MS only after other possible factors that might be causing the symptoms are ruled out.

The diagnostic procedure in general is thus a three-part process. First, the patient's medical history must be taken and evaluated. Then comes the most important part, the neurological exam. Finally there is lab work.

Let's have a look at all three.

THE MEDICAL HISTORY

The first thing neurologists will wish to do when a patient arrives for an initial visit is to take a complete medical history.

Every doctor has his or her own style of going about this job. Some do it formally, instituting a standard series of tests and queries. Others are more casual in their approach. They start by asking leading questions and then listen carefully to the response. A simple inquiry such as "How come you're here today?" can sometimes be enough to get the ball rolling. At other times patients may have been dragged to a doctor's office by their families and are reluctant to open up. A doctor might handle this situation by simply saying, "You don't really want to be here, do you? Well, since you are, why don't we try to get to the bottom of this thing that's bothering you." The variations are endless.

Personal style notwithstanding, there are basic facts that physicians will wish to bring to light, especially if MS is suspected. The following list, typical of what a neurologist might ask during a first interview, is worth taking mental notes on before the initial visit, with an eye toward being properly prepared, and as a means of helping physicians come to a more rapid, effective assessment.

• When did you notice the first symptoms? What were you doing at the time? What happened that caused you to take note of these complaints? Describe how they felt.

• How often do the symptoms appear? Do they come and go intermittently, or are they constant?

• What seemed particularly strange or atypical about the symptoms?

• In what ways—and at what rate—have the symptoms progressed? Have they changed in any noticeable way over the past weeks and months? How?

• Do the symptoms hurt? In what ways? How often, and at what times of day or night do they bother you? If pain is present, what helps relieve it? Has the pain gotten worse or better since you first became aware of it?

• Can you recall having had similar problems in the past? Is it possible that you have experienced these same symptoms before and did not pay attention to them at the time?

Physicians will question patients concerning their general health:

• How would you characterize your present state of health? How has it been through the years? Do you consider yourself a healthy person? Why or why not?

• Are you suffering from any diagnosed chronic ailment? High blood pressure? Arthritis? Asthma? Diabetes? Heart problems?

• What type of surgical operations have you undergone during your lifetime? Have you had surgery of any kind recently? If so, what was it for? Describe the procedures at length.

• Do you have allergies of any kind? Are you taking medications for them?

• As far as you know, do you have an allergy to any specific drug? If so, which ones? Have you had any serious reactions to drugs in the past?

• Do you smoke? If so, how many cigarettes a day? How long have you been smoking?

• Do you drink? How much, and how frequently? Do you habitually take drugs or tranquilizers of any kind? Have you ever been treated for addiction?

• Do you exercise? What kind of exercise do you practice, and how frequently do you do it?

• Describe your diet. What is your attitude toward nutrition in general? Do you tend to eat a lot of fats? What kinds of fats? Do you monitor your cholesterol frequently? What is your present cholesterol level?

• Have you ever suffered a serious vitamin deficiency? Were you treated for it?

• How well do you sleep? Have you experienced sleep problems over the past few years? If so, describe them.

Although at the present time there is no known etiologic relationship between multiple sclerosis and toxic on-the-job pollution hazards, a doctor may wish to gather a certain amount of background concerning a patient's occupation:

• What is your present job? Where do you work? What do your duties entail?

• How long have you been at this job? What previous employment have you held over the years?

• In what ways, if any, do the symptoms you are complaining of interfere with your work? How recently have you noticed these changes?

Childhood and family history are especially important:

• Where were you born? How many years did you live in the place of your birth? Did you move before you were a teenager? From where to where? Exactly how old were you when you moved?

• What is your racial or ethnic background? Where did your ancestors come from?

• Did you suffer any major physical problems as a child or teenager? Any major accidents or operations? Describe them.

• Do neurological diseases of any kind run in your family? If so, which ones? Which relatives have suffered from them?

• What was the general health of your mother and father? Did they suffer from chronic diseases of any kind, such as diabetes, circulatory problems, or MS? Are they presently alive? If deceased, what were the causes of their deaths?

• Do any of your family members now have a neurological disease? If so, describe their condition: how long have they had it, what degree of seriousness has it reached, and so forth.

Psychological and emotional modalities will be probed:

• How do you feel psychologically and emotionally? Have any major life problems recently emerged? Have you experienced any type of emotional trauma in the past year or so, such as a divorce or the death of a loved one?

• Have you been depressed lately? Did the depression start for a particular situational reason, or is it the free-floating kind?

• Are you under a good deal of stress at home or at work? In which ways does it affect you?

• Have you noticed any sudden changes in your emotional or mental state lately? If so, describe them. For example, do you find yourself crying more easily than usual? Have you experienced anxiety attacks or feelings of listlessness or despair? Have you noticed any changes in your ability to think clearly?

• Have there been any recent and dramatic changes in your memory or memorization capacity? How is your attention and concentration?

• Have you ever been treated for psychiatric problems? If so, describe them.

A person's present state of health will be profiled:

• How is your appetite? Any changes in your eating patterns?

• What is your weight? Has it changed dramatically up or down in the past six months?

• Do your bowels move regularly? Have you noticed any change in regularity over the past few weeks or months? Have you recently experienced constipation or other elimination troubles?

• Are you prone to frequent urinary problems or bladder disturbances? If so, describe them. Do you feel an increasingly frequent need to urinate? Are you ever—or have you ever been in the past—incontinent?

• How would you characterize your everyday energy level? Have you noticed any alteration or drop in this level? Any dramatic changes?

• Have you experienced any problems with your vision lately? If so, describe them. Do you have frequent headaches? Eye pain? Blurred or double vision?

• Are you in pain of any kind?

• Have you recently experienced strange, bizarre, or peculiar symptoms? Describe them. Are they intermittent? Do they come and go, or do they remain relatively constant?

• Do you experience difficulty of any kind walking, making sudden turns in direction, or getting in and out of a chair? Any coordination difficulties? Head or facial pains? Changes in your handwriting? Dizziness? Shaking? Numbness, nausea, loss of feeling, or a pins-and-needles sensation anywhere on your body?

The above list represents a sampling, of course, and physicians will each have particular questions they prefer to ask, many of which will be tailored to a patient's age, sex, physical condition, and presenting symptoms.

Note that some of these questions appear to have little to do with neurological disease per se. There are several reasons for this. First, most doctors like to obtain as complete physical and emotional pictures of their patients as time and circumstance allow. Second, a majority of patients come to a doctor's office complaining of symptoms, not of a particular disease, and it becomes the doctor's job to ask a series of wide-ranging questions to narrow down the field of possibilities. Finally, in the course of such an interview patients will often divulge seemingly inconsequential bits and pieces of information about themselves that later turn out to be major aids in achieving a diagnosis. One neurologist has made the following interesting observations on the importance of such seemingly secondary information:

The most significant thing you can do for a [neurological] patient is to spend time taking a medical and personal history. It has to be documented if you're going to get a total picture and deal with the person as a whole person. I like to know things such as, was there anything wrong with their birth? Was it prolonged? Was it a toxic birth? Did their mother have difficulty carrying them? What has life been like in general? Where have they lived most of their life? What kind of infectious diseases have they had? Have they ever been jaundiced? What kinds of diseases run in their family?

I don't know what this has to do with things, really, but in my records it gives me bits of information, threads that I can follow through a person's life. For instance, I have a patient who developed Parkinson's disease at age sixty-five. He's a psychiatrist who lives in an old Victorian house in Orange County where he sees his patients. This man tells me that for years people have been coming into his office and saying they smell gas. Finally, he had the gas lines checked and, sure enough, leaks were found. So I started wondering: Was there a relationship between this man's condition and the many years he spent inhaling the gas? Perhaps there was. Perhaps, I told myself, I should pay more attention to this line of reasoning.

Then there's another patient I've followed for years who has developed rigid hypokinetic parkinsonism. Some time ago he and his wife went camping for a week in a cabin in Maine. It was the middle of the winter and they were using a propane stove to keep warm. One night they fell asleep and the gas escaped from the stove. The man woke up, dragged himself and his wife through the door, but by the time they got outside she was already dead. The man then spent a long period of time in the hospital recovering. Now, propane gas poisoning causes hypoxic changes in the brain, and it is a well-known fact that carbon monoxide can produce a clinical syndrome that looks like Parkinson's disease. Today this fellow stoops, shuffles, has a slight tremor, suffers from obvious bradykinesia. In other words, he has what appears to be Parkinson's disease. Was the condition caused by the gas? I'm not sure. But if I hadn't found out about this exposure I would certainly have had a lot less data to go by when I diagnosed him.

THE NEUROLOGICAL EXAMINATION

After the medical history has been taken, doctors will conduct a thorough physical and neurological examination in order to home in on the particulars.

They will be anxious to know, for instance, where in the body symptoms are located. In a typical case of MS, assume that a patient presents with a patch of trouble in the optic nerve, a patch in the cerebellar connection between the legs and arms, and a patch in the spinal cord, affecting the legs. This picture represents trouble spots in three different parts of the body which, in a tall person at any rate, can measure as much as a foot apart from one another.

The doctor must now consider what ailment might cause the appearance of three seemingly unrelated symptoms spaced so far apart.

MS, it turns out, is one of the most likely candidates to produce several simultaneous areas of nervous-system abnormality. In fact, its most distinctive characteristic is that it affects multiple sites. This is why it is classically talked of as being "disseminated in time and space." "Time" here refers to the history of the patches of trouble as they have expressed themselves—disseminated themselves—over the years. "Space" refers to the nervous system itself, where the symptoms tend to be located—disseminated—several inches or even several feet apart from one another and/or from the original source of trouble in the nervous system. Evidence of dissemination in time and space is always grounds for suspicion of MS.

Elements of the Exam: What to Expect

The eyes will be examined, usually with the aid of a colored grid called an *Amsler chart*. Patients will be asked to focus on a red dot in the center of the chart. If they have difficulty seeing this spot (recall that a dark hole in the center of one's vision is a possible indicator of MS), the eye is then examined for signs of pallor along the optic nerve. If such signs appear, this means trouble in the optic nerve.

Both the appearance of the eyes and their movements is important. Is one eyelid drooping? Both? Are the eye movements well coordinated? When a patient glances sideward, does one eye move properly while the other seems sluggish and fails to travel as far as it should in the direction of the nose? Since there are relatively few nervous disorders that produce this behavior, such a problem is a strong indication of MS.

The patient may be told to focus on the tip of the doctor's finger or on a flashlight, and the movements of his or her eyes will be observed. If anything unusual shows up, a special striped cloth tape two feet long by three inches wide will be run by the patient's eyes, and he or she will be asked to count the number of stripes. While the counting goes on the doctor looks for nystagmus, repeated jerking movements of the eye. Patients may also be told to look in a certain direction as the doctor examines for spontaneous saccades—rapid intermittent eye movements. In general, the eyes will be looked at extremely carefully if suspicion of multiple sclerosis is present.

Hearing will be tested too, but the doctor ordinarily does this in the course of the exam by speaking to the patient in a conversational tone and observing the response. If the patient appears to have trouble hearing, the doctor may talk in a purposely low tone or even whisper to gauge the degree of the defect. Voice quality, amplitude, speech, and tone are assessed in a similar way, by listening to the patient speak and noting any slurring, blurring, or arrhythmic voice patterns.

The patient is now told to walk across the room, perhaps on the pretext of picking up a folder or stepping on the scale, so that he or she will not self-consciously—or unconsciously—try to disguise a gait or coordination problem. Sometimes a slight limp, hesitation, wobbliness, or drag in the foot will be seen.

When MS is suspected doctors will always be on the lookout for spasticity. Patients may be asked to sit on the examining table where the doctor lifts one of their knees. In a normal patient the knee assumes a jackknife position. In a person with stiffness or spasticity, the leg extends straight out for a moment, then goes limp.

At times the only way spasticity becomes apparent is when patients perform a series of complicated movements. They may be asked to walk briskly across the room, bend over, pick up a book from the floor, straighten up, turn around, sit in a chair, stand up, then sit down again. In the process stiffness in the legs may be noted, a jiggling motion or bounciness of the gait. But not always. In the early stages of MS spasticity tends to come and go, and can rarely be produced on demand. Only when a person is performing the most complex physical maneuvers will it be noticeable (skipping or running is a good test; the legs can often be seen brushing awkwardly against each other when MS involvement is present). Young patients with plenty of stamina may be asked to perform jumping jacks or pushups, hop on the ball of one foot, run in place. Occasionally a patch of trouble in the corticospinal pathway will reveal itself through such strenuous activities.

Strength and coordination are tested. Patients will be asked to resist pressure, such as pushing against the doctor's arm. Or the patient will be told to make specific movements such as alternately patting the front and back of one hand with the other in rapid succession. This is an excellent gauge of coordination and cerebellar function. (It is also, interestingly enough, used as a gauge of mental acuity by some doctors: the faster the hands are able to move back and forth in succession, the theory goes, the higher the intelligence.)

Hypotonia will be looked for. For example, a patient is asked to sit on the edge of the examining table while one of the knees is tapped with a reflex hammer. In normal persons the knee kicks forward once with a short jerk, then comes to a rapid stop. When hypotonia or lack of tone (remember that tone is the muscle's ability to resist an applied force) is present, the leg jerks out and then continues to swing back and forth several times like a pendulum; there is little or no muscle tone present to slow down its movement. When performing the knee-reflex test, persons with MS may also kick forward violently, an example of *hyperactive reflexes* and a sign that a patch of trouble exists somewhere on the main controlling pathway from the brain to the spinal cord. This response is especially indicative of MS if it is accompanied by stiffness.

An equivalent method exists to test hypotonia of the arm. A patient extends an arm, the doctor grips it at the wrist and instructs the patient to pull the arm toward his or her face. The doctor resists the movement for several moments, then suddenly releases it. In normal people the hand will snap backward several inches towards the patient's face and then automatically stop. With hypotonia the hand continues moving swiftly backward without any dampening effect to check it, sometimes to the point of bouncing off the patient's face.

The *Babinski* or *extensor plantar reflex* is one of the best-known neurological reflex findings. Here the doctor rubs the outside edge of the patient's sole with a reflex hammer or any blunt instrument, and watches for a normal downward inflection of the toe. When the corticospinal tract running from the cortex of the brain to the spinal cord is affected, the toe will do the opposite of what it does with a healthy person, flexing upward instead of down.

If the Babinski is extremely abnormal, the whole leg will react: the ankle will flex, the knee bend, and even the hip may show some degree of flexion. In patients with advanced spinal-cord disease this reflex can be so sensitive that when a tongue depressor or reflex hammer is brushed lightly across any part of the foot, even the top, it will trigger a wildly uncontrolled flexing reaction.

A patient may also be asked to touch a finger to his or her nose. If a peculiar side-to-side tremor is observed while the finger approaches the face, the accumulated experience of neurologists indicates a patch of trouble in the cerebellar connections to the arm.

Since MS patients tend to lose their abdominal reflex, this reaction is routinely checked. With the patient on the examining table, the doctor scratches lightly on the person's belly with a sharp instrument such as a wooden tongue blade. In a normal patient the stomach undergoes a slight muscular contraction. Persons with MS often display no reaction at all.

One must, of course, consider the entire picture when an

abdominal reflex is absent. One woman patient, for example, had been through five childbirths, several of them prolonged. Though she showed no reflex reaction when the blade was passed over her stomach, her lack of response was in fact due to the thick stretch marks that had formed across her abdomen and were preventing her from feeling the pressure of the blade. The same can be true for obese patients or for those with thick scars on their stomachs from surgery or wounds.

On the other hand, a young person with a normal-sized stomach usually has no problems reacting to the abdominal reflex test *unless* a neurological condition is present. Occasionally, the only indication at all of MS involvement will be lack of this response. Sometimes this is all that is needed to suspect MS involvement.

Patients will be given sensory exams. One of the most common is the *joint position sense function test.* Patients are told to place their feet together and shut their eyes. Normally, when examinees are deprived of vision they will receive enough sensory information from their joints to tell them where they are standing, and to keep their balance. If they consistently break station and lose balance, this is a probable sign that some degree of sensory dysfunction is present in the joint position sense.

A similar test consists of having patients close their eyes, and quizzing them on whether their big toes are extended up or down. The doctor then moves the toes and asks if they can identify the new positions.

One of the most useful sensory perception challenge tests consists of measuring a person's ability to perceive tactile vibrations. Various grades of tuning forks are used, the most common vibrating at cycles of 128 or 256 cycles per second. The tuning fork is tapped and set in motion, its strength of vibration set appropriate to the patient's age (an older person will be less sensitive to vibrations than a younger person, and will require a stronger vibration). The fork is touched to some part of the body, usually a toe bone, knuckle, or tip of a finger. If the person's vibratory perception is intact he or she will clearly identify the moment when the vibration stops. If not, neurological trouble is a possibility. Electronic versions of this test are also used.

Other sensory tests include the following:

• *Ability to perceive temperatures:* An examining physician places his or her hands on a patient's cheeks. In a normal person the doctor's hand will seem to radiate approximately the same degree of warmth on both sides of the face. A substantial discrepancy perceived by patients between the two sides can hint at some type of sensory abnormality.

• *Awareness of sharpness test:* Using a pin or broken tongue blade, the doctor lightly jabs different parts of a person's skin. In cases of sensory deficit a particular area will feel the jab less acutely than others, or sometimes not at all.

• *Tickle sensation:* Using a feather or a piece of rolled-up tissue paper, the doctor strokes the patient's cheeks or forehead. Patients should feel approximately the same pressure and sensation on both sides of the face.

Mental function is checked. Although some doctors seek this information by administering written mental-status exams or asking patients a set of predetermined questions, it is more often accomplished by means of ordinary conversation. During the examination, for instance, doctors will ask questions that a mentally alert person should be able to answer without trouble, questions pertaining to the patient's address, the day of the week, the morning's weather, and similar matters of common knowledge. Patients may be asked to do an unchallenging mathematical calculation, or to spell simple words. Even politics may be discussed, with the doctor probing to see if the patient knows simple things like the name of the current president of the United States. Conversing in this way, the doctor quickly obtains a rapid picture of the patient's memory, orientation, alertness of mind, and thought organization.

During the physical exam the entire body will be checked. Many doctors start at the top and work down.

First, the skull is examined and palpated to determine if it is inordinately small or large or if it contains hidden bumps or lumps or even old scars from past operations. (One patient who claimed never to have undergone surgery was found to have a large brain-surgery scar hidden beneath her thick hair. She had simply forgotten about the operation, it turned out, a possible sign in itself that a mental deficit of some kind was at work.)

The face is examined. Is it expressive? Symmetrical? Patients are asked to make a repetitive sound such as "me, me, me!" The doctor observes how well the lips move and how evenly the voice rhythm is maintained.

The gag reflex is checked to see if the throat contracts and elevates in a normal way. Then the head is rotated and the neck arteries listened to with a stethoscope for noises, called *bruits,* a possible sign of trouble.

In the upper extremities the arms are examined to ascertain if any differences in the size of the muscles exist or to see if one arm is shorter than the other. The heart, lungs, and abdomen are all given a routine check.

As we have seen, sexual dysfunction is a possibility in MS. Thus, if the patient complains of trouble in the groin area, especially numbness in the perineum, a detailed examination will be made.

The *bulbocavernosus reflex* will first be tested by squeezing the vulva or penis. The bulbocavernosus is a muscle that ensheathes the "bulb" of the penis in males, and the bulbus vestibuli in females. Under normal conditions these areas produce a reflex contraction of the anus when squeezed. If there is a patch of trouble at the bottom of the spinal cord where the nerves from the perineum connect to those of the anal sphincter, the reflex will be absent or considerably slowed. For males the cremasteric reflex will also be assessed by scratching the inside of the thigh and observing if the testicles retract upward in a normal way. Other tests can be made in this area as well.

Finally, down to the lower extremities. Here the doctor is looking for bulk, tone, strength, coordination, and facility of movement in the legs and hips. The patient is asked to stand barefooted and to tap his or her toe rapidly on the floor. The tendon reflexes of the legs are checked, a Babinski reflex test applied, and a general examination made.

By now the entire mind and body have been given a thorough medical once-over, and a great deal of information has been gathered concerning both a patient's state of health and the possible cause of his or her symptoms.

The last pieces of the picture will now be supplied by lab tests.

LAB TESTS

When a neurological examination presents evidence of MS but the examining physician does not feel entirely confident in the diagnosis, the next steps will be taken in the laboratory.

Here the most likely tests include a CT or CAT scan (computerized axial tomogram) or, if the local hospital has one (which it often does not owing to the high costs of this machine), an MRI (magnetic resonance imaging). Evoked potential tests will probably be on the agenda as well, plus several blood tests.

Let's have a look.

CAT Scan

Of the two most frequently used imaging devices, the CAT scan and the MRI, the CAT provides an older and less sensitive technology. Developed in the early 1970s, in its time it represented an enormous improvement over standard tests such as angiography, not only because it took clearer pictures and involved a faster procedure, but because the strength of the X-rays themselves were considerably less powerful, and hence less potentially harmful, than those used in prior technology.

Run by a computer imaging system known as *computer tomography*, the CAT scan beams X-rays through a patient's brain at different angles and densities via a rotating scanner, which then produces numerous cross-sectional computer images of the examined areas. These are studied and evaluated in three-dimensional pictures on a TV screen.

Capable under certain conditions of picking up lesions, tumors, and sclerotic plaques, the CAT scan is just as likely to miss these telltale indications or to produce ambiguous images. Thus, while the CAT scan was the favored imaging technology of the 1970s and early 1980s, today the MRI has become the machine of choice whenever it is available.

The MRI

Run by an electromagnetic mechanism so large that its generator must often be placed outside the confines of the hospital building in a separate kiosk, the MRI is a highly sensitive magnetic imaging machine capable of locating plaques not only in the brain but in the brain stem and, to a limited extent, in the spinal cord as well. When used on the same patient over a period of many months, it can track his or her progress, locating plaques when they emerge (especially those grouped in the ventricular areas of the brain, where MS lesions commonly form), or noting the fact that no new plaques have developed since the last MRI was taken.

The technology that runs MRIs is straight out of *Star Wars*. Lying on a platform called a "scanner bed" inside a narrow spaceship-like capsule, patients are exposed to strong, intermittent bursts of a magnetic field that causes hydrogen protons in their tissues to give up their normal random movement, start spinning in unison in the same direction, and line up, as it were, in rows.

A radio frequency signal is then beamed into the magnetic field, which momentarily allows the protons to move out of alignment. The signal is then stopped and the protons return to their rows, in the process emitting a discrete amount of energy. This energy is read by a magnetic receiver coil within the MRI, measured, and the information is transmitted to a computer, where the data is transformed into crisp, three-dimensional TV-screen images of the tissue areas scanned.

When undergoing this test patients will first be positioned onto the scanner bed, where straps and a head cradle are set in place. Then the scanner bed is moved into the magnetic tube.

Inside the tube odd noises occur, especially the banging sound of the radio waves turning on and off. The patient will be asked to lie perfectly still for a half hour to an hour and a half, depending on the amount of computerized data required. Afterward the images will be analyzed by an MRI specialist. Occasionally more pictures will be required during a single session, and the patient will be asked to return to the capsule for further studies.

At the present time there are no known health risks involved in using an MRI. Unlike X-rays, magnetic fields appear to cause neither short- nor long-term ill effects. Yet, although in nine out of ten cases magnetic resonance will locate the areas of trouble, the machine is not 100 percent accurate, especially in finding spots on the spine and brain stem, and it cannot be counted on to provide absolutely conclusive evidence of MS involvement. Moreover, although patches of trouble may be seen on the MRI screen, there is often no guarantee as to whether they are MS plaques or lesions caused by other diseases. Sometimes, as well, several strenuous sessions inside the cramped MRI must be undergone before a full assessment can be made.

MRIs are expensive, though an increasing number of insurance plans cover them today; and, as mentioned, the machine is so costly to purchase and install that many—most—hospitals in the United States do not have them on hand. Moreover, the tubelike capsule that patients must lie in when being screened can be frightening, and in cases of severe claustrophobia the lesser powers of the CAT scan will be preferred. For people who are uneasy over the prospects of a tight fit, a tranquilizer can be asked for before the session begins. If patients have a metal part inside their bodies, moreover, especially a pacemaker or shrapnel from an old wound, these objects can be damaged and even moved around inside the patient's body by the MRI's powerful magnetic field. (One patient had recently had a large amount of dental work done, including the fitting of several metallic plates; when exposed to the magnetic field in the MRI she complained that she had difficulty keeping the dental plates from coming off and flying out of her mouth!)

Evoked Potential Tests

As we have seen, when the neural pathways running throughout the body are damaged, the disordered areas interfere with the normal impulses that transmit command messages from one part of the nervous system to another. Evoked potential tests (EP) are designed to measure these impulses, and to detect discrepancies in their transmittal. Such discrepancies can be caused by tumors, they can be signs of simple inflammation, or they can be the result of sclerotic plaques.

Three types of EP tests are currently in use:

1. The *somatosensory evoked potential test* (SEP) assesses the flow of nerve energy from the arms or legs to the brain.

2. *Brain-stem auditory evoked potential tests* (BAEP) scan the nerve pathways from the ears to the brain, using earphones that emit repeated clicking or tonal sounds.

3. *Visual evoked potential tests* (VEP) monitor nerve conduction from the retina to areas of the brain in the occipital lobes, which are responsible for sight. VEP testees are seated in front of a TV screen that displays a color-changing checkerboard grid. One eye is covered and optic response to the changing patterns is recorded.

These three tests are administered by attaching disk electrodes to sections of the scalp, the location of each electrode being determined by the sensory systems under examination.

Pulsing electrical signals are then sent through the electrodes, and the nerve reactions to these mild shocks are measured and transformed into oscillating waves on a computer screen. The wave forms are then studied by doctors and lab technicians with an eye toward ascertaining the time lapse that occurs between the electrical stimulation and the nerve response. Any problem detected in the continuity of nerve flow is possible evidence of impairment along the nerve pathways.

EP tests take from a half-hour to two hours to administer, depending on how many areas of the body must be tested. Occasionally, the shocks transmitted by the electrodes are irritating.

But not often. In ninety-nine cases out of a hundred, EPs are painless. If after analysis, signs of nerve-impulse impairment are discovered, and if these signs agree with evidence of plaques already seen on the CAT scan or MRI, a diagnosis of MS will be strongly indicated.

Or, in another scenario, a patient may be found to have a single spot of trouble on the spinal cord, yet complain of several symptoms in different parts of the body. If the EP is performed, hitherto unknown patches may be discovered that help to confirm the diagnosis. In general, the MRI and EP complement one another, and when similar results are found in both this fact is ordinarily considered ample indication of MS—assuming, of course, that the medical history and neurological examination support these findings.

Lumbar Puncture

If the results of both the neurological examination and the lab tests are thoroughly analyzed but continue to remain uncertain, doctors may seek further information by ordering a lumbar puncture test (LP).

Popularly known as a spinal tap, the LP was once the terror of patients in hospitals throughout the land, primarily because of the supposed pain factor involved. Today, thanks to improved technology, the LP is a relatively painless process routinely ordered for a variety of possible ailments. The procedure is simple. With patients sitting on the examining table or lying on their side with legs pulled up in fetal position, an area on the lower spine is cleaned and anesthetized. A hollow needle is then inserted between two of the vertebrae and a test tube's worth of cerebrospinal fluid withdrawn. (The cerebrospinal fluid is the watery substance that surrounds, cushions, and protects the brain and spinal cord.) The test takes from twenty minutes to a half-hour to administer.

While an LP alone rarely provides proof of MS, it supplies critical information about a patient's body chemistry that adds substantially to a doctor's knowledge base.

For instance, if patients show signs of unexplained cellular materials in their spinal fluid such as lymphocyte-type white blood cells, this indicates that inflammation or infection is present, and is grounds for further investigation. Normally, lab technicians expect to see several lymphocytes in a spinal-fluid sample. If ten or twenty appear, this is a typical sign of MS. Certain types of immunoglobulin, specifically the IgG variety, are also elevated in MS patients, and their presence adds further corroboration to the picture.

After spinal fluid is withdrawn, it will ordinarily be submitted to an *electrophoresis test* to determine if abnormal blips of protein, known as *oligoclonal bands*, are in evidence; in more than four-fifths of MS patients they are. A combination of elevated lymphocyte count plus abnormal proteins and/or immunoglobulins is a formula that is highly suggestive for MS.

Blood Tests and MS Look–alikes

At the present time no definitive blood tests exist for MS. And yet blood tests are an important tool in the diagnosis process as a means of *excluding* other diseases whose symptoms resemble those of MS (a crucial element in the diagnosis of MS, you will recall, is diagnosis by exclusion).

Take, for example, vascular disorders. When a person's small blood vessels become so inflamed that they interfere with normal blood flow, multiple patches of trouble can be produced that strongly resemble certain symptoms of MS. Lupus erythematosus is one such disease.

Other types of infections that can mimic MS include syphilis, AIDS, certain cancers, and a handful of viruses. Indeed, the similarities between these diseases and MS turn out at times to be so close that doctors may follow patients for months, even years, and never be entirely certain whether the person has multiple sclerosis or a look-alike disorder.

To rule out many look-alike ailments, therefore, blood tests have their place. Blood will be drawn, smears taken, and a variety of possible tests performed. When the results are in they will then be added to the patient's file of information, and a final diagnosis will be made.

At least, it will *usually* be made.

WHEN A DIAGNOSIS IS DELAYED

In certain cases, especially when clinical and laboratory findings are negative or inconclusive, a diagnosis may be put on hold. In a few situations there may even be a question as to whether any pathology at all is present. Quirky, unexplained symptoms do occur at times. They come, they annoy, and they pass, never to return.

In other instances doctors may be unclear as to whether the problem is MS or a look-alike disorder. In still others, only inconclusive hints can be found during the neurological exam, and nothing positive shows up in the lab tests, even though the patient is clearly symptomatic. Under such circumstances a physician will be forced to take a wait-and-see approach.

Don't be surprised, for instance, if you are called back at a future date for more testing. Or, if after waiting several weeks, you are informed that the results of the exam are inconclusive, and that you must schedule another appointment several months down the line for further assessment. Important to note is that since MS is disseminated in time, two or three examinations spaced out over several months will often fill in the missing blanks and clinch a diagnosis. Let's say, for example, that during the first visit the doctor finds signs of a cerebellar side-to-side tremor in the right arm. Stiffness and hyperactive reflexes are also in evidence, but nothing definite is determined. Then, during examination number two, the tremor is gone but a hole in the vision, a *cecocentral scotoma*, shows up on the Amsler chart. The patient also has slightly slurred speech at this time, and some loss of sensation in the left arm.

Now, if the neurologist finds that after several visits the patient's symptoms continue to change in this characteristically MS-like way, this fact can be one of the most persuasive we have for reaching a diagnosis. It demonstrates that:

1. A look-alike disease such as lupus or cancer is impossible. None of the look-alike disorders mentioned above behave in this erratic way.

2. The symptoms observed are all typical or possible complaints of MS.

3. The fact that the symptoms change dramatically from month to month, and that such changes are a characteristic of MS, is a powerful piece of evidence to support a diagnosis.

These changes, when observed over time and viewed in the larger context of the exam and lab results, can eventually point directly to MS, if not with absolute certainty, then certainly with a substantial enough degree of probability to reach a final conclusion.

Finally, in a last-case scenario, doctors may simply be stumped, telling patients the somewhat disconcerting news that as things stand there is no way of coming to a definitive conclusion, and that right now waiting and watching is the best—and only—strategy.

Still and all, and despite the possible delays that occasionally attend the diagnosis, in most instances patients will learn what their situation is a short time after the examination and lab tests are completed.

Then, assuming it *is* MS—what now?

4

Dealing with the Diagnosis

So you have MS. What now? To begin, it's a given fact that different people react to the diagnosis of a serious disease in a variety of ways. Let's have a look at some of the most prominent of these reactions, with an emphasis on the difficult ones, and learn what can be done to cope.

DENIAL—ESPECIALLY FOR THE CAREGIVER

The doctor is wrong, the patient thinks. What do all those tests prove, anyway? I'll seek a second opinion. And a third, and fourth, if necessary, till I get this thing straightened out. Ralph R., an MS patient for more than twenty years, recalls his early reaction to diagnosis:

> I never wanted to go to the doctor at first and my mother and sister had to schlepp me through the door of the waiting room. Most of the time I thought this whole thing was a bunch of garbage. I had some eye trouble and a bad hip, that's all. Why the big deal? After going through

the examination and all, the doctor called me in and told me I had multiple sclerosis. He starts to go through all these things I should and shouldn't do, and I remember, I blanked on him inside. I didn't listen. I put up a barrier between him and me. I didn't know what MS was, and I didn't care what it was. I wanted to go home. When my sister and mother asked what the doctor said I told them I had a disease called multiple sclerosis. They got very excited and messed up. "What the hell's wrong with you!" I yelled at them. "What the hell do the doctors know!" They asked me what I was going to do now. "What do you expect me to do, stand on my head?" I shouted. I was real hostile and didn't want to face any of it.

Denial is a normal human response to loss. People experience it when they are fired from a job, when they receive a setback in business, when a loved one becomes terminally ill. The archetypical example, perhaps, is the person who loses a beloved husband or wife, then continues to talk to the deceased as if he or she were still alive.

People who receive bad news tend to process it in stages. First comes the shock: "What? Me? MS!"

And the denial: "No, not me! Not MS!"

Then anger: "Why me?"

Followed by depression and desolation: "Poor me!"

And finally, acceptance: "Yes, me."

Though these stages do not necessarily follow one another in neat rank and file, and while they sometimes come all at once or in alternating patterns, they *do* come for just about everyone diagnosed with a chronic disorder. It thus becomes the job of friends and family to help the stricken person sort out these feelings, to work through and talk through this twist of fate until the affliction is accepted. Eventually it will be.

In some ways even, denial is a healthy defense mechanism. It allows the unconscious mind time to sort out painful realities, to ponder the problem, and to come up with acceptable accommodations. It is not necessarily a harmful process, at least not in the beginning.

But there are dangers. These become evident when denial continues for prolonged periods of time, when a patient insists that there is nothing to worry about, that he or she needs no clinical help or advice, that nothing, absolutely nothing, is wrong at all.

Following a serious medical diagnosis, such an attitude can be especially harmful. Persons in denial postpone returning to the doctor for follow-up treatment. They turn a cold shoulder to medications and therapy that might improve their condition. In time the symptoms worsen and discomfort comes; but still they insist that all is well, that everyone is getting worked up over nothing. Difficult as it is to believe, there are cases of persons with MS who have become bedridden, yet who continue to maintain that the problem is simply a bad back or virus attack, and that they will soon be on their feet again.

The best medicine for denial is time. Time, plus honest discussion between family members and an open, receptive relationship between patient and doctor. When family members bring up the matter of a loved one's diagnosis they would do well to emphasize the "glass is half-full" approach. Stress the fact that MS tends to frequently go into remission; that most MS patients lead full, active lives; that medications will relieve discomfort; that MS does not involve pain; that some people recover entirely. Help the person confront the reality of the situation, but do it gently, with tact, never trying to ram the truth down the person's throat.

In most cases denial is a stage in a process that has a beginning, middle, and end. In most cases it will pass, giving way to a let's-get-on-with-it, let's-deal-with-it attitude. Just give it time, space—and loving support.

ANGER AND DEPRESSION

Another possible negative reaction to diagnosis is anger: "Why me?" the patient says. "I'm young. I was healthy and happy yesterday. Today my life is ruined! I'm no good to anybody, and nobody's good to me!"

This anger aims in two directions: at others, and at oneself. In both cases persons suffer. Though the famous pioneer of thanatology, Dr. Elisabeth Kübler-Ross, once remarked that the answer to

"Why me?" is "Why not me?"—for the fact is that millions of people develop chronic diseases every year—telling this to patients affords them cold consolation at best. Better to simply let the person's stormy transaction with the world unfold as it will, trying not to take the anger and negativity personally in the process. Like denial, it will pass in time.

The danger to watch out for here is that anger can become the central emotion in a person's life, and that the patient will seem to undergo a kind of personality change because of it, becoming uncharacteristically irritable, negative, and reactive to harmless things said and done by others.

Can these reactions be caused by the disease? Once in a while, perhaps. But most likely they are a response to learning that one is chronically ill, or to the despair that follows.

What can the patient *and* caregivers, family, and friends do to get themselves and their loved one through this rocky period of time? Try the following:

For the family: When faced with a barrage of angry, disruptive behavior on the part of a newly diagnosed person, family and friends will be forced to confront their own resentment. The first impulse felt when a son or daughter, husband or wife, boyfriend or girlfriend starts acting in new and difficult ways may be to storm out of the room or even deliver a right hook to the jaw. This is an understandable reaction, and a human one. In the face of an already problematic situation, however, family members are advised to bite their tongues, swallow a few times, and keep their cool. Screaming scenes only produce more screaming.

- When and if you become exasperated to the point of blow-up, don't play the martyr. Escape temporarily. Go to a movie. Exercise. Visit a friend. Refresh yourself. Then come back and try again.

- At times the best approach to angry patients is to confront them in calm, supportive, but decidedly direct terms. Say how sorry you are, and that to the best of your ability you sympathize with their plight. But you are finding it difficult these days to cope with certain aspects of their behavior. Identify these behaviors,

being careful to choose your sentences carefully. Avoid ul-
timatums and negatively charged buzz words such as "always,"
"constantly," and "terrible." Phrases like "Your screaming is
making me crazy" or "I just can't take this anymore" are better
left unsaid. A little goes a long way here. Suggest that you talk
about these problems, that the patient verbalize what he or she is
feeling, and that both of you try to work things out together.

This is tricky, of course, and the circumstances must be right.
Studies have shown that people are most receptive to new ideas
and heart-to-heart talks during comfortable times of day, such as
at the dinner table or in the evening before bed. Avoid making this
attempt when you are angry, or when the patient is bothered or
preoccupied. *Especially* avoid them when both of you are in a sour
mood or in the midst of an argument. As a rule, however, a
forthright, well-timed confrontation can clear the air and get
things back on an even keel.

For the patient: Persons who are caught up in distracted, long-
term angry states are often the last ones to know about it; their
behavior at times is largely unconscious. It thus behooves them to
look for telltale signs. Typical of these are:

• When one finds oneself picking fights with others over petty
issues.

• When friends and family members consistently complain
about the patient's moods; or when they repeatedly tell the patient
that he or she is "not acting like himself or herself anymore."

• When friends one ordinarily sees on a regular basis stop
coming around.

• When petty annoyances set one off into prolonged, petulant
moods.

• When a person feels increasingly withdrawn and isolated
from friends and loved ones.

All the above can be danger signs. Again, one must consider
the fact that a diagnosis has put you temporarily into a negative

state. This is to be expected. Just be careful that the negativity doesn't get out of hand, or that you don't hurt others while processing out your own problems.

If you are feeling particularly hostile toward the world, and if things show no signs of getting better, outside help may be in order. A section on psychological and social resources is included in a later chapter.

Learning that you have MS is a bitter pill, especially if the symptoms cause dramatic changes in your body and in your lifestyle. So go ahead and mourn. Mourning has an important place in the process. But after you've mourned and processed it through to the best of your ability, let it go and determine to make the best of what fate has handed you.

Easy words, perhaps, but necessary ones. It has been determined time and time again that MS is a disease that is directly influenced by a person's state of heart and mind, and that a positive attitude toward one's condition has positive effects not only on one's outlook but, most likely, on one's symptoms as well. Depression, despair, anger, all come with a built-in stress factor that may very well make things worse, certainly on a psychological level and, many experts believe, on a physical one as well. A number of resources are out there to help you come to grips with this matter, some closer than you think. In a later chapter we will deal with this subject at length.

DIGESTING THE NEWS—STEPS YOU CAN TAKE RIGHT NOW

"What now?" you ask yourself. What about my parents, my girlfriend, my boyfriend, my children, my boss? How will they respond to the fact that I have a chronic neurological disease? Will I become a burden on them? Will I lose my job? Will my disease progress quickly? Will I be able to afford the medical bills? How will I adjust to this change in my life? Where do I begin?

You begin at the beginning, by allowing yourself the opportunity to digest the news of the diagnosis.

Start by awarding yourself quiet time alone to weigh the situation, to process it, to feel it, to face it. Discuss it with your friends, or with family, clergy, doctor, therapist, anyone who listens well and whose advice you trust.

During this period of adjustment stick close to the status quo. Now is *not* the time to buy a new house, to look for a new job, to take a trip around the world, or to burn your bridges. All—or some—of these things will come in due time. For the present simply let the news percolate inside you; allow yourself the luxury of quiet consideration, and of thinking ahead.

Perhaps your first inclination is to get a second opinion. Is this wise? Unless you have good cause to think that your diagnosis is flawed, unless you are thoroughly unhappy with your doctor and have solid medical reasons to doubt his or her diagnosis, why put yourself through more of the same?

This is not to say that second opinions should inevitably be avoided. Sometimes they are necessary, but only if there is legitimate reason for seeking them. The fact is that most neurologists know their stuff and tend to be highly accurate in their clinical assessments, especially when backed up by advanced laboratory technology. If you have any doubts, discuss them with your doctor first. If your doctor cannot resolve these questions, he or she will more than likely be willing to refer you to another specialist.

Above all, bear in mind that panic and despair are blind alleys, and that if you throw in the towel in the beginning others around you will do the same. In most instances, MS is a manageable disease. In fact, the odds are good that you have brushed shoulders with other MS patients from time to time in your life and not even known they have the disease. So take stock, try to get yourself on an even keel, and plan on making the best of things.

In the meantime, the same question arises: What to do at the present time?

As is often the case, the best way to start coping with a difficult new reality is to deal with the things you can do *right now, this very moment*. Ask yourself:

• What steps can I take to prepare for the future, both the long-term and short-term future?

• What problems may arise? How can I prepare to meet them?

• What information do I need? Where can I find it? What are my resources? Which ones will I need right away?

• What are my immediate needs and goals this present day, both medical and personal?

If possible avoid the "can'ts." You will think about them another time. Better to mobilize the "cans" and put them to work right away. Emphasize your assets and abilities, your strengths and resources. Deemphasize worry. Put fear on hold—it restricts and restrains. Stress action, practical coping measures, and positive thinking. These will help you through. Here are some experience-proven suggestions, strategies, and caveats to get you started.

Learn All You Can About MS

First, get all the information you can from your doctor, especially in the beginning. Compile a list of important questions and bring it to your next appointment. Any doctor worth his or her salt will be happy to sit down with you and help you establish your options. But remember, physicians are busy men and women and sometimes need to be prodded. Don't assume they will volunteer everything they know on the subject of MS, or that they will magically intuit your needs. Sometimes they won't. Take the bull by the horns: ask.

Meanwhile, be careful of hype and hearsay, of canned information and two-week miracle cures, of superficial newspaper articles and five-minute specials on the ten-o'clock news. Far better than falling victim to half-truths is to learn everything you can about multiple sclerosis for yourself, so that you will not be vulnerable to false claims, and so that you will be able to pick and choose your resources from a position of knowledge rather than fear.

Educate yourself. Read books and newsletters on the subject

of MS (see Bibliography). Ask questions, talk to medical professionals, attend lectures, clip articles, keep a notebook, go to the library, borrow audio and video tapes on MS, seek counsel from other patients. Send for literature from MS organizations, especially the National Multiple Sclerosis Society (see Appendix for addresses). They are a veritable cornucopia of free and valuable aids. Last but not least, if the spirit moves you, attend an MS support group in your area. These organizations are a spectacular source of knowledge and sympathetic support for many people, patients and families alike. It is well worth at least one visit to such a group to find out if it suits your needs. It most likely will.

Don't Judge Your Situation by That of Other MS Patients

Every person with MS is different. This is an axiom that should be kept constantly in mind. No two MS patients are ever exactly alike.

Don't suppose, for example, that because Mr. X has trouble walking you will have trouble walking too. You may or you may not. Or that because Mrs. Y is taking a certain medication you will need the same. It may not be appropriate for your needs. Some people will develop a symptom, be treated for it, and the symptom will not show up again for thirty years. Others will have the same symptoms for the rest of their lives. The process is unique for every individual. It can't be second-guessed.

A corollary to the above is that you cannot necessarily know the future of your condition from the past. To a patient who has experienced multiple sclerosis for several years and is expressing fears about the years to come, it can be pointed out that, well, you've had the problem now for six years. It's true that during this time your symptoms have become more troublesome than they were at the start. You can't get around as well as you did awhile ago. All things being equal, the chances are that in another five or ten years you will be a little more disabled than you are today. But this is only a possibility. The amount of disability a person will or will not develop is unknown. It may be more, it may be less. There's no way of predicting it with certainty.

Unpredictability is intimidating, of course, yet it cuts both ways. On the debit side, it means you must live with an ongoing question mark, perhaps for the rest of your life. That's a tough job. But in the asset column this very unpredictability gives hope. Remission can come at any time. Symptoms may never return, or they may plateau out at a certain level and remain there for decades. One or two exacerbations may occur and then never recur. And so forth.

A diagnosis of MS, in other words, in no way "dooms" you to a predictable and progressive decline, as a diagnosis does in many other chronic ailments. You are, as it were, in the hands of your own particular fate.

Hear MS patient Joseph De V. on this subject:

> I was fortunate when I first developed MS to have the help and kind words of my uncle, who suffered a case of the same disease. Both of us had what you'd call a mild case of MS. We both function well and have not had to take many medications. At first I looked around and went to a support group. I didn't go back for a long time after because of what I saw there, a lot of persons in wheelchairs with caretakers. People all crippled up. I got terrified and forgot to notice that a lot of the others looked normal. I talked to my uncle. He said that the same thing happened to him, not at a support group but seeing a film about MS that scared him out of his wits. It was full of advanced cases. A nurse he knew told him not to worry, that only a few people ever get this way, and that every person who has MS is a separate case. You can't predict your own condition by others. It's not the kind of thing you can know. Anyway, I took this to heart and remembered it when I got depressed. I kept telling myself that I was me, not them. What happened to them was their problem. What happened to me would be different. You take your chances; you hope for the best. Prayer never hurt either.

Know Your Resources

There is presently no cure for MS—but there are many things you can do right away to manage the disease. Perhaps a cure for

MS will be discovered. Perhaps. Until that time it is futile to torment yourself with hopes, to hang on to every tabloid claim of an imminent wonder drug. The hard fact is that even if an effective remedy for MS was developed tomorrow residual effects would probably remain, and these could very well continue to cause some degree of dysfunction.

It is far better, therefore, to concentrate on the resources and aids at hand.

For example, chemotherapy exists that will help relieve symptoms and exacerbations. A wide variety of drugs are available that can be used to palliate such symptoms as spasticity, balance disorder, facial neuralgia, urinary infection, fatigue, depression, and others. Physical therapy in many cases has proven an effective aid to MS sufferers. So have home exercise regimes. Many varieties of counselors and medical professionals are available to help patients cope with psychological and social needs. Good nutrition, vitamin regimes, relaxation techniques, and many other self-help aids exist. Don't hesitate to use them. You will find many of them mentioned throughout the pages of this book.

Good Quality of Life Is More Important Now Than Ever Before

When MS patients become sick they tend to suffer flareups and to feel more uncomfortable than they might if they did not have the disease. Consequently, it is more important now than ever to take good care of yourself and to nourish your body like a doting parent. Approach this task in a determined, multidimensional way. A later section of this book will be dedicated to an in-depth look at what you can do to improve your general state of health. The following suggestions will get you started:

• Get plenty of sleep. Determine how many hours a night it takes to make you feel refreshed, then stick to this routine faithfully. Burning the candle at both ends is highly discouraged for MS people. There is, it might also be mentioned, some anecdotal information that MS persons are at their best in the morning. Early to bed, early to rise may help.

• Without pushing beyond your limits, get plenty of exercise, activity, fresh air, the works. If your condition allows, take a brisk walk each day. Follow a calisthenics regime at home, preferably one tailored to your needs by a medical professional. Even if you are wheelchair-bound there are exercises that will get the juices flowing. We will profile these in a later chapter.

• Eat a well-rounded diet. Keep the intake of various "problem foods," such as fats, fried foods, and sweets, at a moderate level. If vitamins seem to make you feel better, by all means use them.

• Watch your bowel movements. MS persons tend to get constipated. This is normal, but it should be monitored. If there are signs of chronic constipation and if you tend to go long periods between movements, talk to your doctor. Impaction must be avoided at all costs.

• If you smoke, try to give it up right now. It will do your condition no good, and it may make things worse. Smoking, as you no doubt know, plays a prominent part in a number of cardiovascular diseases. Why put more of a burden on your system than it is already carrying?

• Stay away from narcotic drugs, especially stimulants such as amphetamine or cocaine. They are pure anathema for all MS sufferers. Drink moderately, if at all. Although alcohol in small amounts is believed to have no adverse effects on MS, temperance is always a wise course. If you already suffer from balance problems, moreover, one drink too many can trigger a fall. If you have a tremor, alcohol will occasionally make it worse. Excess alcohol can interfere with sound REM sleep, and persons who rely on it to relax find that over time it worsens their feelings of restlessness and dis-ease. Be cautious in this department.

What about caffeine? Mild tea and soft drinks are okay for most people, but be careful of coffee. It is a diuretic, and diuretics increase the body's urine production. If you already suffer from bladder disorders such as frequency or urgency, coffee will increase your need to urinate even more. Best here to experiment, find out what effects coffee and other stimulating drinks have on your condition, weigh the pluses against the minuses, and act accordingly. Your goal now is to strengthen your immune system and to become as healthy and fit as circumstances will allow.

Learn Your New Physical Limits and Stay Within Them

MS is not a disease that tolerates being pushed. If you try, you may end up flat on your back. The disease is extremely unforgiving in this way.

As a result, it makes no sense to force yourself to perform physical activities that every fiber of your body is resisting. This does not mean, of course, that one should make no efforts at all. Far from it. But once you discover how much you can do in a day, and how long it takes to do it—after you have discovered your natural endurance limits and tested them out—it is sound policy to abide by these guidelines and not let your reach exceed your grasp. A few hints in this direction:

• Find out what your best times of day are and get the majority of required work accomplished during this period. Are you a morning person? An afternoon person? An evening person? Experiment. Test. Once you have discovered your peak times map out the day accordingly.

• In the workplace, the same rule applies as above. If you know you have X amount of work to do, plan to do it in those hours when your functioning is highest.

• When exhaustion overcomes you unexpectedly, don't resist it. Rest until it passes. This is important. Pushing when you are overtired and enervated is a dangerous mistake.

• Slow and steady is best. Avoid rushing or trying to cram everything in at once. Studies in the workplace have shown time and again that employees do the best work when they pace themselves, and when they work at a comfortable, methodical rhythm.

• Set realistic goals at the beginning of each day. Some people write down each item they hope to accomplish. They take this list to work or post it around the house as a reminder. Then, if fatigue overcomes them at some point during the day and they fall short of the mark, they still have several items on their list checked off and do not feel so frustrated.

• Don't get discouraged if you must stop an activity in the middle and postpone finishing it till later. If you fail to get everything done today you will do better tomorrow. Make this resolve a motto for yourself; the resolve itself will often be enough to keep you positive.

• Become more relaxed and philosophical about your accomplishment needs. There is, after all, only a certain amount of work each human being can do in a day, and this depends entirely on one's storehouse of energy. If chronic disease has reduced your storehouse, this is simply the fact of the matter. It is not your fault, and there is certainly no need to beat yourself up about something beyond your control. As fully as you can, come to terms with this realization. In the end you will find that by accepting your energy limitations you will lead a more satisfied and productive life.

Learn to Identify Problem Situations and Devise Methods for Avoiding Them

There are a number of everyday situations and conditions that can bother MS patients. Get to know the ones that personally affect you, and whenever possible work around them. Some of the most common are listed below:

Heat

A classic reaction in most MS patients when exposed to extremes of heat is a worsening of symptoms, and sometimes a recurrence of old symptoms. Possible danger situations include taking a sunbath or a hot shower, lolling in a hot tub or sauna, running a fever, or simply suffering through the dog days of an August afternoon.

Reaction to heat is so endemic to MS that at one time it was even used in making the diagnosis: Patients were placed in hot baths and any MS-like changes in their neurological functioning were noted. (It has also been found that MS persons who suffer from scotoma and who are placed in a hot tub for thirty minutes or more show an immediate increase in this vision problem when tested on the Amsler chart.) Though such tests are no longer necessary, persons who suspect MS should pay attention if exposure to heat makes them weak and exhausted, and should report this fact to their physicians.

Why does MS react adversely to heat? No one is certain, though it is known that heat reduces the speed of impulses along the nerve pathways and thus slows an already impaired system of responses. Fortunately, the effects of overheating are transient, and when patients enter a cool environment the symptoms tend to dissipate. What can you do to counteract the effects of heat? Try the following:

1. Air-condition your home and car, especially if you live in a hot climate. Keep the receipt after you buy the air conditioner too. Any appliance or device that can be shown to have a therapeutic effect on an MS person's condition is usually tax-deductible. Some MS people even deduct a certain amount for the air-conditioning portion of their summer electric bill, though this one can be tricky.

2. Steer clear of steam baths and saunas, exposure to sun in an open place such as a ballpark or beach, going outdoors during the hottest hours of the day, or putting yourself in situations where you know you will become overheated, such as in crowded rooms or busy public places.

3. Don't sunbathe enough to work up a sweat. When you go into the sun wear a scarf or a hat with a brim on it. Walk on the shady side of the street. Stay well hydrated and drink plenty of cool liquids when the weather is hot (though not necessarily iced). Take frequent rest stops in shaded doorways or under trees as you go. Wear thin, loose-fitting clothes in summer, and open-topped shoes like sandals (the feet serve as a kind of thermostat for the entire body; when they are cool the rest of the body tends to be cool too, and vice versa). Shop in air-conditioned stores, or better don't shop at all on very hot days. Avoid crowded places and non-air-conditioned public transportation. When you have outdoor work, get it done in the cool hours of the morning and late afternoon. Or confine your labors to overcast days. Some MS persons take the Oriental route and carry parasols or umbrellas with them during the steamy summer months.

4. When you take a bath or shower, be careful not to get overheated. Don't soak too long. Keep water temperature at a moderate heat only.

5. When you have a cold or flu, be careful of fevers. The higher the thermometer goes the more likelihood there is of a symptom flareup. The best medicine here is prevention. Be careful of exposing yourself to family members with colds and flu, and take extra precautions during the winter season when viral infections are rampant. When you are exposed to contagion stay warm, eat properly, get quality periods of sleep and rest, drink lots of liquids, avoid crowds, and wash your hands frequently.

When you do have fever use aspirin or an aspirin substitute such as acetaminophen (Tylenol, Datril, Anacin-3) to keep temperature down. Acetaminophen is less harsh on the stomach than aspirin and produces few if any side effects.

6. Dr. Louis Rosner in his book *Multiple Sclerosis: New Hope and Practical Advice for People with MS and Their Families* reports that during the hot months of the year some MS people find that aspirin helps manage symptoms produced by excess heat. According to Dr. Rosner, patients report that this simple trick prevents such MS-related disorders as fluctuation of vision. Dr. Rosner also suggests that when persons become overheated, soaking their legs in cold water helps lower body temperature.

7. If you become suddenly overheated during the hot months, impromptu methods for getting the body temperature down include dunking in a pool or sprinkler (preferably in the shade), taking a cold bath or shower, wiping oneself down with a wet sponge, sucking on ice, and using wet compresses, towels, and ice packs. Running cool water over the wrists for three or four minutes is an old cooling-off trick that works for many people. In India people suck on a lime when they become overheated. Fanning also helps.

Cold

Although cold tends to have a less harmful effect on MS symptoms than heat, it should be avoided under certain circumstances.

Supercold baths, for instance, are not a good idea. In fact, any extremes of temperature should be avoided, and this includes alternate cold and hot baths taken to treat back and muscular problems.

On January days, cold temperatures can have a slowing effect on the muscles of the arms and legs, and walking on ice is always a problem for persons with balance and gait disorders. Extreme cold tends to irritate the eyes of some MS persons.

Unlike heat, however, cold has its place in MS therapy. Patients generally tend to feel their best on cool, crisp days, and a temperate climate in general is conducive to improved well-being. Cool baths can do much to mitigate the effects of overheating, and iced gel packs help relieve the muscle spasms and stiffness brought on by spasticity.

For people with numbed sensitivity of the throat, moreover, a standard therapy known as "thermal stimulation" relies entirely on cold temperatures to stimulate improved reflex response. A laryngeal mirror (or any long, safe metallic object) is cooled in the refrigerator, then placed at the back part of the throat for several minutes. If this routine is repeated several times a day over a period of several months, the cumulative effects often help restore some degree of sensation and reflex response to the mouth and swallowing muscles.

Crowded, Confusing Environments

Some MS patients find that busy places and mobbed social scenes make them anxious and unfocused. For persons with balance difficulties the jostling of crowds can be risky business. Those with vision disorders find driving at night or in heavy traffic to be problematic. Persons with bladder disorders may feel that excusing themselves from a social gathering every few minutes to use the bathroom is embarrassing; after a while they simply choose to stay at home.

But assuming that you are on your feet, there is no real reason to stay at home. Instead, schedule activities around your specific limitations.

If confusion is a problem, for instance, socialize with small groups rather than large. If loud gatherings seem overwhelming, stick with smaller, intimate affairs. When you are socializing in a crowd, avoid speaking to several persons at once. Simultaneous verbal input coming from different directions can be distracting to MS people. Stay with one conversation at a time.

Pick and choose your recreational spots. If you bowl or play golf, and assuming your condition permits, go on the off days or nights of the week when fewer people are around. Pick relatively quiet, uncrowded places to get together with friends: a small restaurant, a neighborhood pub, your own dinner table.

Avoid malls and shopping complexes on weekends and holidays when the crowds are heavy. Shop at supermarkets in the off morning hours. Don't drive during peak traffic times. Leave for work at an earlier hour to avoid traffic snarls. If you take a bus or subway, travel during the off times. If you commute regularly to school or work, carpool and let others do the driving.

During the Christmas season it may be expedient to send a relative out to do your shopping for you; or you may wish to shop by mail. If you live in a city and enjoy excursions, choose times of day when the streets and parks, museums and theaters, are the least populated. Students can schedule classes at convenient times of day that best suit their needs. If they run into the usual scholastic rules and scheduling regulations, they should talk to the office of student affairs or the dean of students; the administration of schools and universities are now obliged, both ethically and in some cases legally, to make special arrangements for disabled students, especially if they are walking impaired.

Those who walk to work should consider taking a shorter, less crowded route. Parents who take their children to a playground are advised to find a play area that is off the beaten track and that has plenty of benches for sitting down. Take rests whenever necessary. Plan ahead.

You don't, in other words, have to severely curtail your comings and goings when you have multiple sclerosis. Simply live and have fun in ways that place less pressure on you while you're at it.

Fatigue

Fatigue is a major problem among MS persons and limits almost everyone at one time or another. Thus the suggestions given above apply here as well. Don't push yourself. Learn to live within the margins of your energy quotient and plan your activities accordingly. Avoid taking on more tasks than you can handle. Budget your time. When you are tired, rest. When you are forced to abandon a project because of exhaustion, pick it up later at your convenience.

There is, of course, also a psychological side of the fatigue issue. Mary P., a nurse with MS, talks on this theme:

You get so you can't get around like before. That, let me tell you, can get you down. It's frustrating and can drive you crazy. You feel useless to yourself and others. You stand at a crossroads. You have to say to yourself, I may be impaired to some extent but there are lots of things I can still do. You say that, or you say "I give up." Of course, giving up isn't very smart, especially when you don't have to. I gave up for a while, but then got my act together and started making the best of things. One of my main problems is that I get tired easily. I said to myself, if I get tired I will not be embarrassed to tell others about it or to excuse myself for a while. If they don't like it, that's their problem. They know I have MS. They can stretch a little. It doesn't hurt them a bit. At home I have asked my husband to help out, and he's been great. I still do plenty of the chores, only I do them more slowly. I do things like heat up TV dinners instead of cooking big meals. I am working part time now, and thank God my legs are okay. Nursing is a demanding field, but so far I've been able to keep up. If someday I become too weak to do it I'm preparing myself now for that ahead of time, so that when the time comes I can exit from the job gracefully.

Much work has been done over the past years, especially in the field of occupational therapy, to help MS patients feel better about themselves by learning to apply tricks and shortcuts that neutralize the problems of fatigue. Occupational therapy (OT) in general is a field dedicated to showing persons how to adapt to their disabilities in a maximum way, and to help them deal more easily with the everyday tasks of daily life. In later chapters we will discuss a number of OT techniques as they specifically pertain to weakness and fatigue.

Avoid Dangerous or Difficult Situations

Another critical part of determining physical limits is to arrange activities in such a way that potentially hazardous, embarrassing, or daunting situations are avoided.

For example, if you are walking or balance impaired, it is imperative to think in terms of ambulation safety. A protruding lump on the stair carpet can become a deadly tripping machine for persons unsteady on their feet. An ungraded walkway leading to the front door can send a person sprawling. When driving a car not specially equipped, drivers may discover their brake foot has suddenly cramped or gone weak.

Again, it is a matter of planning ahead. Start with your own house or apartment. Locate all potential hazards, both inside and outside; either eliminate them entirely, or modify them for your needs. In a later chapter methods for accident-proofing the household will be fully discussed.

Plan out your walking or driving routes in advance, and stay off dangerously congested roads. If night vision is a problem, drive only during the daylight hours. If special prescription glasses are needed, keep them on your person at all times.

Patients with urinary urgency should schedule comings and goings so that a bathroom is always within a reachable distance. Persons who fatigue easily should have a plausible excuse and "escape route" planned out whenever they socialize or attend a public function. Persons with swallowing difficulties must avoid all foods that cause choking, even if this means revamping one's diet.

Another good plan-ahead idea is to keep a fully stocked first-aid kit in your home in case of accident, being sure every few years to resupply old or outdated medications. This doesn't mean you must run out and buy an expensive prepackaged kit, although if you can afford it it's not a bad idea. It does mean there should always be a stock of standard items somewhere in your house just in case. A well-supplied first-aid kit contains the following items, all of which can be purchased at a local pharmacy:

Bandages and sterile gauze pads
Tourniquet stick and wrappings
Roll of adhesive tape
Elastic Ace-type bandages
Cotton and cotton swabs
Razor blades
Knife
Needle and thread
Matches
A candle
Tweezers
Safety pins
Scissors
Cough syrup
An antihistamine
Aspirin and/or aspirin substitute
Baby oil and mineral oil
Calamine lotion
Petroleum jelly plus any favorite salves and ointments

Epsom salts

Smelling salts or ammonia (for treating unconscious persons)

Antacids

Iodine or any good disinfectant

Rubbing alcohol

Hydrogen peroxide

Eye drops (check with your doctor for the best ones if you have eye problems)

Diarrhea and constipation medications

An emetic (such as syrup of ipecac)

Hot and cold packs

Oral or rectal thermometer

A pen, paper, and flashlight

A good book on first aid

Also important are phone numbers, such as those of your doctor, dentist, neurologist, a local poison control center, police, fire department, ambulance, and address of the nearest emergency room. Some people tape important emergency phone numbers on every phone in the house.

Caution and carefulness are more important now than ever. The idea is to cut down on the elements in your life that cause accidents or embarrassment by simply avoiding them from the start.

Work Closely with Your Doctor

If you have MS, chances are that you will continue making frequent visits to a physician as time passes. There are several reasons for this.

First, since MS symptoms tend to change over the course of time, your doctor will need to see you on a regular basis to assess the nature of these changes, and to deal with them medically.

Second, if a diagnosis is in doubt, several consecutive visits will reveal information that a single examination cannot.

Third, as different primary and secondary problems arise, new medications will become necessary. Sometimes dosages must be modified and different medicines tried out. Referrals to other medical professionals such as physical therapists may be necessary as time passes.

Fourth, staying in touch with your physician is simply smart practice. Doctors and their staffs can be a source of ongoing support and assurance. They can provide advice when it is asked for, reassessment when it is needed, and referrals if secondary complications arise. Regular attendance at a doctor's office can prevent worry and instill peace of mind. If you have a problem, don't stay at home and let your imagination blow it up out of proportion. Get it checked.

A good relationship between physician and patient is thus a central part in the battle against multiple sclerosis. It is, in a sense, a kind of marriage that will last for many years, with both partners being called on to contribute their share of input. So don't be shy about seeking your doctor's help. Ask questions. Keep medical phone numbers close at hand. Feel free to contact your doctor whenever you need advice, or whenever you think that a symptom needs attention. If for any reason you feel that a physician does not meet your standards, if he or she seems uninformed about MS, if your questions go unanswered or ignored, if you constantly feel rushed or forgotten in the office, and if you do not believe you are receiving adequate medical treatment, especially in times of crisis, it may be time to look around for another doctor who will better suit your needs.

When You Need Help, Ask for It

Realize that there are many medical, social, and psychological resources out there that can help in dozens of ways—right now.

The list starts with physicians. From here it goes on to include mental-health counselors, occupational therapists, social workers, home aids, physical therapists, visiting nurses, speech therapists, nutritionists, menu planners, chauffeur services, plus a number of government agencies that specialize in helping the disabled.

Think also about local support groups, group therapy, consumer health-care organizations, newsletters, hotlines and 800 numbers, legal-aid societies, local clergy and community aid, health-care-provider agencies, telephone reassurance services, emergency response systems, medical lending libraries, companion services, neighborhood outreach programs, vocational training, medical referral services, chronically ill day-care centers, respite centers for caregivers, caregiver assistance programs, crisis-intervention facilities, and town, state, and government agencies of all kinds designed to help you get the things you need.

Help is always at hand for an MS person. Know, however, that this help will not always come automatically. You may have to reach out for it at times. But it's there. There are people, both professionals and volunteers, who care, and who really can help in a number of ways. Take advantage of them.

A Positive Attitude Is Half the Battle

It is no longer idle speculation to say that a hopeful, optimistic approach on the part of an MS patient is a kind of medicine in itself. Perhaps it does not hurt to say it again, in red letters: A POSITIVE ATTITUDE HELPS.

Time and time again doctors have noticed that MS patients who maintain a glass half-full rather than half-empty philosophy are rewarded not only with a fuller, richer life but with an improvement in symptoms as well.

Though it is difficult to prove this point scientifically, there are so many anecdotes that point in this direction, such a large number of physicians who have noted it in their offices, and so many, many patients who have found it to be true in their own lives that it can be stated once more that an upbeat, confident, can-do attitude, coupled with a courageous acceptance of whatever disabilities one already has and a willingness to accept what cannot be changed, add up to a better life and a happier patient. We will touch on this point many times throughout this book.

In the pages that follow a wide selection of practical aids, suggestions, and hands-on methods are presented that will help you cope with your malady and add to your general feelings of confidence and control. Up till now we have discussed and defined the problems. In the following sections solutions are provided.

Follow those that apply. If the shoe fits, wear it; if not, find others that do. There is plenty of advice, hints, and suggestions to go around.

In the meantime, do your best to realize that with difficulty comes challenge, and that the act of meeting this challenge with every fiber of your being can in itself be a kind of therapy. Whatever you do, avoid the negatives. Make full use of your resources. Educate yourself and talk to others. Read, discuss, learn, find out. Then deal with the problems that present themselves as best you can. That's all that is expected of you. In a word, strive to remain active, healthy, optimistic, and hopeful. It will help.

GLOSSARY OF IMPORTANT MS TERMS

ACTH (ACTHAR): Adrenocorticotropic hormone. A substance naturally produced by the body which participates in the making of steroids in the adrenal glands, and which is often given as a medication in treating MS. ACTH tends to shorten the duration of time in which MS symptom flareups remain active, although some doctors believe its side effects outweigh its benefits.

AFO: An ankle-foot orthosis. An orthopedic brace that fits over and supports the ankle and lower leg, allowing weavers to walk without a foot drop.

Amantadine (Symmetrel): A medication ordinarily given to Parkinson's disease patients to control rigidity and bradykinesia, but which for unknown reasons sometimes helps improve the fatigue level of MS patients.

Anesthesia: Loss of the sense of touch and feeling occurring in any part of the body.

Ataxia: Lack of coordination in the voluntary movements of the muscles, especially in the muscle groups responsible for reaching and ambulation. Ataxia can cause loss of balance, lurching, staggering, shaking limbs, and impaired coordination.

Autoimmune disease: A disease in which the body's immune system turns against itself and attacks the body's own vital tissues. MS is commonly believed to be an autoimmune disease, and the destruction of myelin tissue (q.v.) is believed to be an autoimmune reaction.

Axon: A nerve fiber that transmits neuronal messages from nerve cell to nerve cell.

Babinski reflex: Response to a neurological test in which the sole of the foot is scratched with a blunt instrument and the movements of the toes observed. In healthy persons the toes curl downward. If the large toe goes up and the others spread apart, this is a sign of spinal tract disturbance.

Baclofen (Lioresal): An antispastic medication given to MS patients to help control spasticity (q.v.).

Brain stem: A part of the lower brain, made up of the medulla, pons, and midbrain, that connects the brain to the spinal cord.

Carbamazepine (Tegretol): A medication used in MS patients to control the sharp facial pains of trigeminal neuralgia (q.v.).

Catheter: A sterile flexible plastic tube attached at one end to a retention bag, used in the catheterization (q.v.) of incontinent patients.

Catheterization: The insertion of a sterile flexible plastic tube called a catheter (q.v.) into the bladder of an incontinent person. Its purpose is to drain urine out of the bladder and pass it down into a bag at the end of tube, thus avoiding wetting and incontinence.

Cat scan: See Computed tomography.

Cecocentral scotoma: A blind spot in the center of the eye, characteristic in MS of disturbances in the optic nerve.

Central nervous system: The combined areas of the brain—cerebral hemispheres, brain stem (q.v.), cerebellum, and spinal cord—which are the neurological nerve centers affected by MS.

Chlordiazepoxide (Librium): A muscle relaxant given to MS patients to relieve anxiety.

CNS: The central nervous system (q.v.).

Computed tomography: Known popularly as a CAT or CT scan, computed tomography testing procedure works by projecting X-rays through the brain at different angles and densities, and analyzing the results of the pictures it obtains with a computer.

Contractures: A painful and disfiguring loss of joint motion caused by several possible factors, including shortening of the muscles and tendons. This condition is often found in bedbound patients who are not being adequately turned and exercised.

Cortisone: A steroid hormone given to MS patients to relieve inflammation and to expedite the healing cycle of symptom flareups.

Dantrolene sodium (Dantrium): A standard medication given for spasticity, usually as a backup or substitute for Lioresal.

Decubitis ulcer: A pressure or bedsore, sometimes appearing on persons who are bedbound or wheelchair-bound. Bed sores most commonly form on the buttocks, back, and limbs as a result of long periods of pressure and rubbing against exposed skin surface areas.

Demyelination: An attack on, and erosion of, the protective myelin sheath (q.v.), which serves as an insulating covering for the body's nerve-cell pathways. Demyelination is characteristic of the disease process that takes place in multiple sclerosis.

Diazepam (Valium): A muscle relaxant and tranquilizer, often prescribed for MS patients who suffer from spasticity (q.v.).

Dilantin: An antiepileptic medication used in MS to control the sharp pains of trigeminal neuralgia (q.v.).

Dysarthria: A speech impairment characterized by an eccentric or broken rhythm of speaking and slurring.

Dysesthesia: Distorted and uncomfortable skin sensations caused by impairment of the sensory parts of the nervous system, especially the sense of touch; most commonly in MS, a low-level uncomfortable and sometimes burning sensation in the extremities.

Evoked potential: A diagnostic machine and procedure used to detect areas of abnormality in the brain which might otherwise remain hidden.

Exacerbation: An attack or worsening of the neurological symptoms characteristic of MS. The word comes from the Latin verb *acerbare*, meaning "to make harsh."

Exercise testing: A process whereby persons are tested for their physical limits and capacity for exercise. Functions such as heartbeat, respiration, blood pressure, muscular strength, motor control, and coordination are measured and evaluated, and the patient is then given a set of exercise guidelines tailored to his or her needs and endurance abilities.

Facial neuralgia: See Trigeminal neuralgia.

Flareup: A worsening of MS symptoms; an exacerbation (q.v.).

Frequency: A tendency to feel a frequent or constant need to urinate.

Glia cells: Supporting cells that repair nerve tissue and act as buffers between nerve cells.

Gliotic plaques: Scar tissue made up of glia cells (q.v.) that forms in various parts of the central nervous system. When gliotic plaques harden they form the sclerotic plaques that characterize multiple sclerosis.

Hesitancy: Difficulty starting the flow of urine.

Ibuprofen (Nuprin, Motrin, Advil): An anti-inflammatory drug frequently given to MS patients to relieve spasticity (q.v.).

Imipramine (Tofranil): A medication given to MS patients to suppress bladder activity and hence prevent incontinence (q.v.). At times it is also given for pain management.

Incontinence: An inability to voluntarily control the process of urination.

Lumbar puncture (LP): A diagnostic procedure in which fluid is removed from a patient's spinal canal and medically analyzed for signs of disease.

Lymphocytes: A type of white blood cell active in the immune system.

MRI: Nuclear magnetic resonance imaging (or testing). Also called an MR or NMR. A diagnostic test in which patients are placed into a narrow tube and a magnetic field is generated through their bodies. The magnetic coils produce certain signals in the brain and spinal cord, which are transformed into computerized images and analyzed for possible signs of central nervous dysfunction.

Myelin sheath: The fatty substance that encases and insulates the nerve fiber, and which is attacked in MS. See also *Demyelination*.

Nocturia: An urge to urinate many times throughout the nighttime hours of sleep.

Nuclear magnetic resonance: See MRI.

Nystagmus: Sudden, jerky movements of the eyes, typical of MS involvement.

Oligodendrocytes: Glia cells (q.v.) from the central nervous system that manufacture the myelin sheath (q.v.).

Optic neuritis: A condition of inflammation of the optic nerve causing sudden and partial loss of sight, usually in the central part of the field of vision.

Oxybutynin chloride (Ditropan): A medication given to MS patients to relieve bladder dysfunction.

Paresthesia: A feeling of pins-and-needles on the skin surface of various parts of the body, a common symptom of MS.

Plaque: A lesion in the central nervous system characteristic of MS.

Prednisone: A steroid drug (cortisone type) used to reduce the tissue inflammation that occurs during an MS flareup.

Range of motion: 1) In physical therapy, a situation wherein a therapist moves or rotates a patient's joints through their full range of normal movements (i.e., rotating a hand 360 degrees at the wrist) as part of an exercise or physical therapy program. 2) In clinical medicine, a situation wherein the physician gauges the degree of motion remaining in a joint, as measured by the patient's active and passive movements.

Retention: A condition in which the bladder does not empty fully during urination, leaving residual amounts of urine, which quickly produce the need to urinate again.

Spastic bladder: A condition in which the bladder fills but does not receive proper voiding messages from the brain. Dribbling, urgency, frequency of urination, and/or incontinence can result.

Spasticity: A condition of increased tone and rigidity in various muscle groups of the limbs and trunk.

Tic douloureux: See Trigeminal neuralgia.

Trigeminal neuralgia: A disorder of the trigeminal (or fifth cranial nerve), which produces sudden, sharp, lacerating pains in the jaw, cheeks, and mouth. An occasional symptom of MS, it is also known as tic douloureux.

Urgency: A strong and sometimes overpowering need to urinate experienced by MS persons with bladder disorders.

Urinary incontinence: A partial or complete inability to control bladder function.

5

Help for the Symptoms of MS

Multiple sclerosis is a manageable disease. This point has been made several times, but it is an important fact and one that all MS persons should keep in mind. A disease, generally speaking, is considered to be medically manageable when its symptoms can be controlled, reduced, and in some cases fully, if temporarily, relieved by medication.

Drugs, however, are only one line of support in an MS patient's arsenal. Supplementing their effectiveness are physical therapy, exercise, rest, health maintenance, occupational therapy, and various self-management techniques, all of which bring symptomatic improvement for a variety of MS-related problems, and all of which are designed to upgrade a patient's level of daily functioning.

In this chapter we will look at the principal medical means that exist for controlling major symptoms of MS. The emphasis will be on the techniques used to bring symptomatic relief *and* on ways MS patients can help themselves in the process.

STEROID TREATMENT

First, let it be said that steroids are complex, sometimes problematic drugs that should be prescribed only when an attack is serious enough to warrant them. For mild flareups, or flareups that come and go in a matter of a few days, their use is inadvisable and most likely unnecessary as well.

In the case of severe exacerbations that last many weeks without apparent sign of remission, however, a brief course of ACTH (adrenocorticotropic hormone) may be prescribed. A hormonal protein produced by the anterior sections of the human pituitary gland, ACTH triggers the cortex of the adrenal glands to increase production of corticosteroid hormones. While technically speaking ACTH is not a steroid itself, it activates steroid production, specifically during traumatic or flight-or-fight conditions such as injury, attack, terror, infection, or intense emotional shock. The type of ACTH used for medicinal purposes is synthetically extracted from animal pituitary.

Originally utilized to treat a demyelinating disease known as post-ineffective encephalomyelitis, ACTH proved highly effective for this purpose, and researchers surmised that it might be of similar value in other demyelinating diseases such as MS. In fact, we now know that ACTH in no way cures MS (though there is some evidence that it aids lesion healing by reducing the number of toxic white blood cells present), but it does speed up the time taken to cycle through an exacerbation. Why this is so is not entirely understood, though like other steroid substances ACTH exerts a suppressing action on the immunological system, lowering antibody production, reducing inflammation, and, it is theorized, disabling those elements of the immune system that produce the MS-causing autoimmune reaction.

ACTH is usually given by intramuscular injection and short-term therapy is the preferred method (long-term use of ACTH is known to be both dangerous and ineffective). The drug is administered in doses of 30 or 40 units daily for a week to ten days, ordinarily under hospital conditions. In most cases flareups subside 10 to 15 percent faster when it is used than in nontreated cases and sometimes sooner. Side effects vary and almost always disappear after treatment ends. Among the possible adverse reactions are gastrointestinal stress (gas, swelling, change of bowel habits, heartburn), acne, increased blood sugar, superfluous facial and body hair growth, puffy face, and high blood pressure. A patient's appetite is stimulated by ACTH injections as well, leading to weight gain, and in some persons a kind of euphoria is experienced, which, to the patient's consternation, tapers off as soon as the drug is discontinued, leaving a depressed "hangover" effect in its wake. The drug also causes potassium loss, and patients are urged to take potassium supplements during the course of medication.

A second and perhaps more medically popular approach to steroid treatment is the use of synthetic anti-inflammatory hydrocortisone medications such as Prednisone, Decadron, or Methylprednisolone. These are usually given in pill form rather than by injection, and in many instances they can be administered on an outpatient basis. Like ACTH, these steroid preparations reduce inflammation, and their side effects tend to be similar to those caused by ACTH.

Exactly how effective are steroid medications for MS? Although these drugs have been used for many years, the answer remains cloudy. Since 1970 when the Schumacher Committee, under the auspices of the National Institute of Neurological Diseases and Blindness, sponsored a multicentered study on the effects of short-term and long-term corticosteroid treatment in MS, there has been little doubt that short-term treatment with ACTH or a synthetic corticosteroid like Prednisone definitely hastens recovery from relapse. This hastening factor is not necessarily dramatic, however, and the beneficial effects quickly diminish after several weeks, with few if any long-term benefits resulting. In the Schumacher Committee study, moreover, it was shown that almost 70 percent of patients who were untreated with steroids improved satisfactorily on their own, and that certain symptoms, such as spasticity and optic involvement, respond far better to steroids than do cerebellar problems such as coordination loss, gait disorders, and tremor.

In some cases, steroid medications do not work at all. In other cases they work only slightly. Treatment is generally most effective during the first few years after a person develops the disease, and as time passes continued therapy produces diminished healing returns. Further, steroids suppress the immune system, putting patients at risk of infection—not simply cold and flu infection but more serious varieties as well. It has also been noted that steroids can produce a potentially dangerous immunosuppressive cycle: Patients take a steroid drug, improvement follows, but when the medication is finished the symptoms return in a matter of weeks or months and more steroids must be prescribed. When the symptoms return, moreover, they are a bit more severe than before. Over time the patient not only becomes dependent on a constant intake of steroids, but the side effects worsen with each course, creating a vicious circle that is difficult to break.

The evidence, in other words, is conflicting. In certain studies, for example, it has been shown that patients treated for optic neuritis with corticosteroids tend to develop MS lesions in other areas of their body *sooner* than patients who do not take these medications. A formal testing of ACTH several decades ago at UCLA under Dr. Augustus Rose evaluated a number of patients who were given intravenous infusions of ACTH, along with a control group given placebo salt solutions. The results of this carefully monitored study showed that patients treated with ACTH indeed improved more quickly than those not treated, though this improvement stopped shortly after the period of treatment was over. But when patients were followed for several months after the study, it became evident that those treated with ACTH returned to the hospital with flareups sooner than those not treated.

Other studies show similarly contradictory data, and at this point medical science is simply not certain as to the long-term value of these drugs. On the other hand, there are many instances where corticosteroids work, and work well, sometimes amazingly well. The side effects of short-term treatment are relatively mild, and in most cases patients indeed report that recovery is faster and easier. Thus, although far from perfect, until a better medication comes along these drugs will undoubtedly remain the first-line drug of choice for the treatment of short-term MS exacerbation.

Finally, while on the subject of steroids, it should be mentioned that certain preparations known as *immunosuppressants* are sometimes prescribed for MS patients, either in combination with steroids or by themselves. Immunosuppressants do just what their name states: They suppress the workings of the entire immune system, especially the lymphocyte white blood cells, the theory being that if the autoimmune process is slowed by reducing the agents responsible for causing it (i.e., the lymphocytes), then myelin destruction will be slowed down as well.

Perhaps the most successful and most frequently used of the immunosuppressants is Azathioprine (Imuran), a substance that has shown some evidence of temporarily reducing the relapse rate among progressive MS sufferers. Cyclophosphamide (Cytoxan) is equally effective in many situations, though its side effects are harsh, occasionally producing cancer in long-term users. Indeed, the side effects of all members of this family of drugs are severe, triggering conditions such as sterility, liver damage, bone marrow suppression, increased risk of infection, and birth defects in pregnant women. For this reason, immunosuppresants remain at the outer circle of the MS pharmacopia and are used largely on an experimental basis.

RELIEVING SPASTICITY

Spasticity is one of the most prominent complaints of MS, and potentially one of the most debilitating. To the doctor manipulating a patient's limbs on the examining table, spasticity presents as an overall feeling of tightness, resistence, and jerkiness, especially in the trunk and lower extremities. Patients, on the other hand, experience it as an enervating stiffness and contraction of the musculature that in mild cases expresses itself as a foot drag, an unbending knee, a hunched posture, or an inflected arm position, in extreme cases as a tightening of the trunk and limbs so severe that it can force a person into a fetal position. The stiffness of the limbs, moreover, makes it doubly hard for patients to go about their daily business, and the extra efforts at movement that must be expended add to the already burdensome condition of fatigue.

Medications for Spasticity

Fortunately, several major antispasticity agents exist to relieve the rigors of this painful and crippling condition. The most effective and widely prescribed is Lioresal (Baclofen), a muscle relaxant that is relatively free of serious side effects and that usually restores flexibility in a gratifyingly effective way.

Lioresal acts at the level of the lower spinal cord and on its descending motor pathways where MS lesions are frequently located. Interacting, it is believed, with the reflex involved in maintaining muscle tone and with the neurotransmitter gamma amino butyric acid (GABA), Lioresal relaxes the main muscle groups in the limbs and trunk, and has an overall inhibiting effect on spasms. This means that if patients suffer gait problems their walking will almost always improve to some extent after taking the drug, as Lioresal works directly on the large muscle groups responsible for ambulation. Physical quickness also improves, as does fluidity of movement and range of motion in the joints. Persons with spasticity of the arms may also experience some gain, though usually less than in the legs. While the ability to move freely and easily will be improved by the antispastic components of the drug, however, related functions such as strength and coordination are not affected.

The dosage for Lioresal is gauged to individual needs. Some patients use it in the morning when they habitually have difficulty climbing out of bed. Later the same day, when the spasticity decreases and they can move without hindrance, the problem lessens and the drug becomes unnecessary. This is an excellent benefit, as continuous action is not required with Lioresal and the drug can be taken on an as-needed basis. After first discussing the matter with one's doctor, therefore, patients are encouraged to regulate the dosage of Lioresal themselves, and to use it only when the need arises.

Patients with spasticity of the lower extremities will usually be started on a low dose of Lioresal, say 5 milligrams taken three or four times a day. This amount will be increased as needed up to 10, 20, or 30 milligrams per dose; most patients respond well within the range of 40 to 120 milligrams a day. Those who require more will probably experience side effects, though some patients tolerate remarkably high doses without reporting toxic reactions. The rule of thumb many doctors follow is to slowly push the dose upward until the drug's full benefits are felt, all the while watching for side effects. If these occur, the dose is then dropped down to a tolerable level. The more significant side effects patients may experience include drowsiness, insomnia, confusion, and generalized muscle weakness, the last being especially problematic, as it can compound the weakness already present in the MS person's limbs (the drug relaxes nonspastic muscles as well as spastic ones).

In general, caution should be taken when using Lioresal if a patient is pregnant, a heavy drinker, has kidney disease or diabetes, or is on other medications such as central nervous system depressants, muscle relaxants, and especially the drug Ethinamate, used to treat insomnia. There is also indication that smoking may interfere with the absorption of Lioresal; tobacco users should discuss this matter with their neurologists if they smoke more than a pack of cigarettes a day.

Another agent commonly used for spasticity is Valium (Diazepam). Though this popular tranquilizer is not as effective as Lioresal for MS, Valium does possess antispasticity qualities of its own and offers the added benefit of being an antianxiety drug, helping patients relax during the day and sleep better at night. Often, moreover, when Lioresal and Valium are taken together, patients report a heightened synergistic effect that is not attainable when either of the two drugs is used alone. While the major problem with prescribing these drugs together is that the drowsiness and weakness, already caused by Lioresal, is compounded, many patients have learned to take this discomfort in stride, reporting that they would rather have their ease of movement restored and feel drowsy than be spastic and wide awake. Others find fatigue and weakness intolerable, and are switched to another medication. Again, determining which drug or combination of drugs is most effective for one's specific needs is a matter of trial and error.

Dantrium (Dantrolene) is a third specific for spasticity and muscle contractions, and as a rule is used only if Lioresal or Valium prove inadequate. Its side effects can occasionally be severe, producing liver toxicity and blood abnormalities. The longer a person stays on Dantrium, moreover, the more likely he or she is to develop problems, and those who take it for extended lengths of time must have their liver enzymes and blood count carefully monitored.

Finally, a general word on spasticity and antispastic medications: although this condition is a debilitating one, there are times when spasticity is actually useful. For example, some MS patients have a limited amount of volitional movement or strength in their legs. For such persons the very stiffness and stubborn resistance of spastic muscles can be an aid rather than a detriment, helping them to keep their legs straight and to stand erect, to pivot, and to transfer without buckling beneath their own weight. Patients suffering from spasticity, therefore, and especially those who have concomitant weakness of the lower extremities, must be carefully assessed when an antispastic medication is being considered in order to make certain they are not being overtreated and hence deprived of a degree of mobility and functioning. In certain cases, especially when spasticity exists in extension of the limbs rather than flexion, antispastic pharmacological treatment of any kind may be counterindicated and may actually make the condition worse.

Physical Therapy for Spasticity

As any MS specialist will agree, spastic patients who fail to request at least one assessment by a PT—a physical therapist—are missing a golden opportunity, as spasticity can often be measurably improved by means of physical manipulation alone.

Interacting with patients on an ongoing basis, physical therapists stretch shortened muscle fibers, increase movement in the joints, and work educationally with patients and caregivers alike, teaching them exercises that can be done at home.

A trained PT will give the patient an initial examination to determine the degree to which their muscle tone is increased or decreased. The physical therapist will pull, push, and generally manipulate the patient's limbs to gauge their level of resistance. One of several formal tests may be used to measure tone and to help determine proper treatment modalities. The therapist will evaluate a patient's strength, coordination, and general ability to perform the daily activities of living.

Once the patient's condition is assessed and the areas of greatest spasticity pinpointed, sustained stretching and body-management techniques are employed to extend contracted muscles, relax muscle fiber, increase circulation, stimulate the sensory receptors in the muscles, tendons, and joints, and return at least some degree of flexibility to the trunk and lower extremities by encouraging the muscles to elongate and detense.

The following manipulations may be used:

• For spasticity of the ankle joint: Either alone or with the therapist's help, patients are told to rise up and down on their toes, extending and exercising the Achilles tendon. Therapists work directly on these problem areas, taking the ankle and leg through a range of passive stretches, and applying gentle but firm twisting and pulling motions to the afflicted areas.

• Range of motion: The therapist rotates the knees, hips, or arms in their sockets, loosening the joints, increasing circulation, restoring elasticity.

• Resistance: The PT pushes on the spastic parts while the patient applies counter pressure, thus extending and exercising key muscles.

• Extension and flexion: With patients lying on their backs, the therapist extends and rotates weakened limbs. Areas worked include the feet, ankles, calves, thighs, hamstrings, hips, lower back, arms, neck, and head. Patients are put into a number of lying, kneeling, or standing positions while these movements are done to maximize the stretch. Patients may also be encouraged to practice these exercises at home with the help of a caregiver. More on this below.

• Manipulation: With patients on their backs, the therapist pulls, rotates, stretches, and manipulates problem areas of the trunks and limbs. Patients with flexed legs or spines may be placed in standing frames and put through weight-bearing maneuvers to encourage postural improvement.

• Movement and exercise: Patients may be instructed to lie on their backs, hug their knees, and rock back and forth to stretch their spines. Bedbound and wheelchair patients are taught stretching and range-of-motion exercises, many of which are profiled in Chapter 6, on exercise.

• Stroking and massage: Slow, purposeful stroking of spastic areas is a standard method for inducing muscle relaxation. General body rubbing and stimulation, deep pressure to the stomach, groin, and lower back, massaging of different spots on the spine, tapping, percussion, all may be used according to the patient's needs.

A special note for caregivers: There are many generic strengthening and stretching maneuvers that can be practiced at home. The following exercises, based on descriptions in the National Multiple Sclerosis Society's booklet *Moving with Multiple Sclerosis* and on advice from practicing physical therapists, represents a sampling that will profit many spastic conditions, and which caregivers can safely practice at home with patients. For more exercises of a similar kind, readers are encouraged to consult Chapter 6.

• With patients either standing or lying on their backs, the arms and legs are rotated through a full 360-degree range-of-motion circle. If assistance is required, caregivers can help move the limbs.

• Patients lie on their backs. Holding a patient's heel with one hand and supporting the area beneath the knee with the other, the caregiver lifts the leg approximately 4 inches up from the bed and pulls it gently to the side for a comfortable stretch. Repeat several times with each leg.

• Patients lie on their backs. Holding a patient's heel with one hand and supporting the area below the knee with the other, caregivers lift the leg several inches from the bed and bend the knee gently toward the patient's chest. Get a good, firm stretch, being careful not to strain or cause pain, then return the leg. Repeat several times with each leg.

• The caregiver holds the patient's heel with one hand and with the other gently but firmly turns the foot to the left as far as it will comfortably go and then to the right. Repeat several times with both legs.

• The caregiver rotates the patient's wrist in both directions as far as it will comfortably go. Repeat several times with both wrists. Massage is applied to the hands. The fingers are gently rotated.

• Patients sit on the floor with legs extended and bend forward at the trunk as far as they can comfortably go. Caregivers kneel behind the patient, place their hands on the patient's upper back, and gently but firmly push the patient's trunk forward, providing a gentle stretch along the entire spine. As the pushing continues, patients can extend their arms, trying (in theory—no straining) to touch their toes. Repeat several times.

Caregivers should remember:

• Exercises should be practiced at least once a day and more if desired. Let the patient determine which exercises are helping and which are not, then proceed accordingly.

• Certain times of the day are better than others for practicing PT exercises. Experiment. Patients will be especially stiff in the morning and may respond better to manipulation when they are up and moving.

• Avoid overheating, overtiring, and overworking.

• Do not work on a patient who is currently experiencing a flareup. Speak with a physician about this.

• Be especially careful when working with a patient who has taken large quantities of steroids, as the potential for osteoporosis and spontaneous bone breaks may be elevated. It is recommended that this matter be discussed with a PT or physician before beginning any type of strenuous exercise.

• All exercises and manipulations should be done slowly. The "No pain, no gain" philosophy does not apply when PT manipulations are involved. Never stretch, twist, or otherwise manipulate a part of the body to the point of pain. If it hurts, you're doing it wrong.

USE OF ORTHOTICS

Another function PTs specialize in is fitting patients for orthotic devices—braces, splints, positioning aids, and ambulatory aids. Here, however, a word of warning. Though drugstores and orthopedic-aid catalogs offer a wide range of orthotic equipment directly to consumers, in the opinion of many health-care professionals it is potentially dangerous to self-prescribe such devices. "The technology of orthotics is changing all the time," says Mary Nishimoto, PT, Associate Director of the Physical Therapy Department at Helen Hayes Hospital, Haverstraw, New York. "You have to really be conversant with these changes to know which ones are best for a given client. There's a lot of room for making mistakes that patients may have to pay for later."

According to Ms. Nishimoto, the manufacturers of off-the-shelf orthotics, in an attempt to make one size fit all, often sell items that end up not fitting anyone very well. "There are so many varieties, sizes, styles, and types of orthotics," she tells us, "that the chance of selecting the best one for a patient's needs is slim, especially if patients don't know much about how these aids are fitted, measured, and worn in the first place. Some patients insist on purchasing the first brace they see in a store or catalog. Maybe they like its color, or the way it looks in the package. Then, a day or so after they put it on, they look down at their foot and find a gigantic blister. They try to take it back to the store, but, of course, since it has been worn the merchant isn't receptive to this idea. So the patient must start all over again and buy another brace that fits better—hopefully."

Poorly chosen orthotics can also place patients in physical jeopardy. "An incorrectly fitted foot brace may cause the wearer to trip," claims Ms. Nishimoto. "It's the same with a poorly matched cane or walker. Incorrectly chosen ambulatory devices put patients at risk of falling. A hastily chosen splint can cut off the circulation and end up being worse than not wearing one at all. There are many things that can go wrong. That's why, in my opinion and I think the opinion of a lot of medical professionals, the best thing an MS patient can do is have a PT or PT assistant fit them for the orthotic rather than choose one themselves. It just makes good sense to take this proven route."

Orthotics come in many sizes and shapes, and again, it takes an expert to know which is best suited to an individual's needs. "These days metal braces are rarely prescribed or recommended," says Mary Nishimoto. "If someone has a foot drop, they should make sure to get a lightweight device made of plastic, one that slips inside the shoe and is worn underneath the pants so that nobody sees it. Also good is a fitting that is molded to the shape of a person's leg. It can be small or very large. It may have a hinge on it, or it may not. Certain styles of orthotics not only support the foot but provide support at the ankle so that the whole leg becomes more stable, all the way up to the hip. But this is not necessarily the best style for everyone. It depends on a person's personal physical requirements."

As with everything, there are tradeoffs. "Orthotic items tend to work very well in general. But there are good sides and bad sides to them. The fact that they get the job done and that they can be hidden from public view is the good news. The flip side is that they can be heavy. Patients sometimes perceive just a few ounces as being a lot of weight to carry. They can be hot in the summer, especially the plastic varieties. Also, it takes a lot of energy to put them on and take them off each time, and MS persons are pretty short of that commodity. Some MS clients have swelling and pain in their feet and can't tolerate wearing shoes and socks. How can such people wear an orthotic too? They can't. It all depends on the individual. This is why having a PT's supervision is so important in the process."

For persons who are new to orthotics, note that the most important telltale sign of a poorly fitting device is the formation of redness over the supported area, specifically redness or chafing that does not disappear within twenty minutes after the orthotic has been removed. Such a condition should be attended to immediately. Prolonged periods of redness can be a sign that there is swelling under the brace or splint; or that the orthotic has not been properly adjusted; or even that the orthotic does not fit at all, and must be replaced. Whatever the cause, don't hesitate if chafing occurs. Sores, blisters, pain, infection, and worse can quickly result.

OCCUPATIONAL THERAPY

For many MS patients, occupational therapy begins in the hospital with an OT consultation, then continues on an outpatient basis and perhaps into the home, where a trained OT visits and makes recommendations for safety and lifestyle modifications. The following helps and hints for coping with safety and ADL factors. Activities of daily living are based on standard OT recommendations, and are chosen for MS persons who suffer from moderate to severe spasticity.

Dressing Aids

The following OT aids for standing, bending, and walking are all useful for persons who suffer from spasticity in the back areas or who are unsteady on their feet. Unlike orthopedic aids, these devices do not need to be specially fitted and can be purchased directly from vendors without fear of safety. (The names of the companies that sell these devices are listed in parentheses after each entry. For addresses see the Appendix.)

• Sock puller—An extension device used for pulling up socks without bending (Sammons).

• Long shoehorn—The grip on this device has a curved handle for easier holding, and its extended length allows patients to put shoes on without bending down (Sammons).

• Elastic stretch shoelaces—Elastic laces allow patients to slip in and out of shoes without constant tying and retying (Arthritis Self-Help Products).

• Shoe and boot remover—Helps to remove shoes without bending down (Arthritis Self-Help Products).

• Dressing stick—All-purpose device for pulling up socks, underwear, pants, what-have-you (Arthritis Self-Help Products).

The following dressing aids help with gripping and arm coordination:

• Zipper pulls—Long-handled hooks provide patients with a broad and firm grip on the zipper. They come in a variety of shapes and forms (Cleo, Sammons).

• Buttoning aids—Though of limited value for many patients, there are a number of different varieties to choose from—loop, cup, hook—one of which may prove helpful (Cleo, Sammons, Abbey, Arthritis Self-Help Products).

More Dressing Hints

Occupational therapists suggest that patients remain seated while they dress. This way the reach down to the feet is shortened and the chances of falling are diminished. It is also suggested that patients dress their weaker side first.

For people with manual-dexterity problems, Velcro tabs make excellent replacements for buttons; many shoes are now available that close with Velcro snaps. Note that loafers are easier to slip on and off than shoes with laces. For a better grip on slippery floors, sneakers, running shoes and bowling shoes are recommended.

Women who have difficulty fastening bras will find front-closure models easier to manage than the back-fastening kind.

It is recommended that patients keep their most frequently worn clothes in the upper drawers of the bureau for easy reach, and that drawer pulls be replaced with large, easy-grip knobs. If reaching up for clothes in a closet is a problem, lower the clothes bar and install the hooks at chest level. If drawers stick and require extra pulling efforts, spray the tracks with silicone or rub them with paraffin wax.

Wear loose, nonbinding clothes that are easy to slip in and out of. Sweatsuits are excellent. So are loose-fitting jerseys, pullover tops, T-shirts, and pants with built-in elastic at the waist. Men who have difficulty buckling a belt should consider keeping a pair of suspenders permanently fixed to their most frequently worn pairs of trousers.

Toileting and Grooming Aids

For persons who are unsteady on their feet, bathroom safety aids such as grab bars and safety rails are a must (Sammons, Abbey, Mature Wisdom). So are nonskid mats and stickers for the tub or shower floor.

Patients with tremors will find electric shavers safer and easier to use than the manual kind. An electric toothbrush or Water Pik may help, as will toothpaste-tube squeezers (Sammons). Sammons also sells a self-rotating toothbrush for persons with limited grip ability. Long, easy-grip handles that fit on shaving-cream cans are available from the same source. Glass drinking vessels should be replaced with plastic or paper cups to prevent breakage. Another useful item is the Little Octopus, a suction-cup device that holds soap to the shower wall or a drinking glass to the sink basin (Cleo).

For persons who have difficulty bending over or keeping their balance while toileting, raised or high-back toilet seats are procurable in a number of sizes and varieties from several dealers (Sammons, Cleo, Abbey). Extension flushing handles are also available (Sammons), along with toilet step stools, splash guards, toilet safety frames, handrails, and toilet-tissue dispenser aids (Sammons). Discuss your needs in this area with an OT or PT before making a purchase.

For bathing and washing, safety is a necessity. Sitting down in the shower is recommended for persons with balance problems; tub stools come in a variety of sizes and styles and can be purchased at any drugstore. Many OTs also recommend bathtub seats. These handy supports come in a variety of models, both the four-legged stool that sits in the middle of the tub, and the flat, clamp-across-the-tub-top variety that adjusts to fit bathtub width. The value of such seats is twofold: they encourage bathers to sit rather than stand while showering, reducing the risk of falls, and they provide easier seating for persons who have difficulty lowering themselves into a tub (Cleo, Sammons, Enrichments). When one is bathing, handrails and safety rails are also a must.

People with unsteady hands may find it easier to trim their fingernails with toenail clippers than standard nail clippers. A nail brush and cloth nail file with suction cups affixed on the bottom are available from Cleo.

Other bathroom and grooming aids include:

• Nail clipper and nail file. These come mounted on a polyethylene board and can be affixed to a wall or tub by means of a nonslip suction cup (Sammons).

• Adjustable extension comb and brush. Both help counteract problems for people with a weak grip (Sammons).

• Long-handled scrub brush. For washing the back and lower extremities without straining or bending (Mature Wisdom).

• Flex-A-Mirror. Easy to set at any angle, with special hand grips for adjustment (Cleo).

• Bath pillow. Supports the head and shoulders when patient is lying in a bathtub (Arthritis Self-Help Products).

• Transfer tub bench. For helping transfer a nonambulatory patient in and out of the shower (Abbey).

• Quad Quip wash mitts. Terry-cloth wash mitts with Velcro wrist closure for persons with limited grip (Sammons).

• Button-controlled shower hose. Easy on/off hand-held shower hose (Cleo).

• Nonslip safety kit. Six 8-inch and six 12-inch self-adhering nonslip safety strips for placement in bathtubs, on shower floors, or on grip railings (Cleo).

Housekeeping and Homemaking Hints

Keep the most frequently used cleaning and household utensils within easy reach. Hang them on hooks, on grids, on shoulder-high or chest-high shelves for easy access. Labels and organization will help: know where things go to save searching efforts. The less reaching and bending patients must do the more energy they will conserve.

The motto used by many MS homemakers and housekeepers is: Adapt, adapt, adapt. For example, if bending makes vacuuming difficult, long-handled carpet sweepers will do the job adequately and demand fewer back contortions. Long-handled dustpans and brooms are also available at most hardware stores. If patients must reach up to dust, dusters can be mounted on long poles. Long-handled dusters are available at hardware stores or through the mail (Enrichments). Persons who frequently move their furniture can put casters on table and chair legs and save themselves the tugging and lifting. Dollies and hand trucks help in this department too, especially for moving heavy objects around a room. A wheeled table known as the Versatilt changes height and angle, and supports up to fifty pounds of household items (Enrichments, Arthritis Self-Help Products).

Persons with an unsteady grip will find that a slip-on handle known as the Push Button Pusher makes it easier to depress spray cans (Enrichments). For one-handed scrubbing, suction scrub brushes adhere to counters or sinks when not in use (Enrichments).

Perhaps the handiest of all household aids is the automatic

extension arm, a long, lightweight plastic or aluminium pole that comes with a lock grip attached to its end and which can be used to procure any small, out-of-the-way item. Just reach for the desired object, depress the trigger at the base of the pole, and the gripper does the rest. Some models include a magnet on the gripper end for holding metallic objects (Arthritis Self-Help Products, Cleo, Sammons, Modern Maturity).

COPING WITH A NEUROGENIC BLADDER

Although a number of patients remain untroubled by bladder difficulties in the beginning of the disease, bladder complaints tend to progress as time passes, specifically for persons with the relapsing-remitting or progressive forms of the disorder. Statistically speaking, approximately three-fourths of MS patients will at one time or another experience at least one form of bladder malfunction, with frequency and urgency leading the list. As with many MS symptoms, the first line of defense is medication.

Bladder Medications

There are two considerations doctors concern themselves with when dealing with MS-caused bladder disorders: management of the social handicaps produced by the bladder difficulties and measurement and treatment of the medical complications caused by the condition.

In the second concern there is little room for maneuvering: drugs and catheterization are the major medical methods used for treating neurogenic bladder. In the first group, however, more latitude exists, and at times—depending on the patient's temperament and wishes—doctors will treat by not treating at all.

For example, certain patients find that for *them* the best method of adapting to frequency, urgency, or incontinence is simply to wear absorbent padded briefs during the day. Psychologically speaking, such persons usually feel little or no stigma about wearing a set of undercoverings that to most of the world is a veritable symbol of infancy and incontinence; they are willing to put up with the wetness and surreptitious changes in the bathroom that such a method requires in hopes of maintaining a relatively normal lifestyle, free of drug therapy, side effects, and catheterization. For patients who are willing to make such a trade-off, this option is singularly well suited. Many MS persons do, in fact, choose the diaper route, especially if their bladder problems tend to be transient, coming and going with their flareups.

For other patients the problem is more complex. For them the mere notion of wearing a diaper is psychologically crippling, arousing images of helplessness, infantilization, and self-soiling. For such persons, it goes without saying, diapers must be ruled out, and medication (or intermittent catheterization) becomes the immediate and necessary means of treatment. A large part of treatment in this area, in other words, depends on an individual's sensibilities and self-image.

When medication is, in fact, appropriate, the doctor must determine what mechanism of bladder disorder is at work. Basically there are two kinds: spastic bladder and flaccid bladder.

Spastic bladder is the more common condition, and the less debilitating. In brief, it works like this: owing to spasticity and muscle contraction, the bladder becomes "small" and fills more quickly than usual with urine. When this occurs, the so-called *voiding reflex center,* a group of nerves situated along the lower spinal cord, send appropriate emptying messages to the brain. These voiding signals are normally blocked by inhibitory messages from the brain until a person needs to void. Demyelination along the neural passages, however, interferes with the brain's "don't void now" commands, and the outcome of this breakdown of communication is loss of voluntary control over the bladder; dribbling, frequency, and incontinence soon follow.

The more serious complication known as *flaccid bladder* results when demyelination forms near or on the voiding reflex center itself. This condition effectively eliminates the center's "voice" that signals the bladder to contract whenever urination is necessary. As a result, the bladder loses its tone, becomes "flaccid," and is unable to empty on cue. The filled bladder soon becomes stretched beyond its limits and finally overflows, causing urgency, dribbling, incontinence, and sometimes, when the urine is pooled for too long a time in the bladder, urinary or kidney infection.

As far as treatment strategies are concerned, the goal is to make the bladder empty more efficiently *and/or* to help the patient cut down on the number of times he or she must urinate each day. There are several useful drugs that help, though a majority tend to be more effective for spastic bladder than for flaccidity.

In some cases, for example, simply taking the antispasticity drug Lioresal, already widely used by patients with spasticity, relaxes the bladder enough so that patients can return to a quasi-normal urinary schedule. But not often. More commonly the anticholinergic drug Ditropan (oxybutynin chloride) will be needed, usually once or twice in a twenty-four-hour time period. In cases of spastic bladder, this drug may be all that is required to keep leakage and frequency under control. One of its major advantages, moreover, is that it can be given on an as-needed basis, meaning that patients can take it to stay dry before leaving the house, then discontinue use when they get home. Ditropan has a narrow therapeutic range before reaching the toxic level, and dosage must be carefully watched.

Commonly prescribed also is Pro-Banthine, an anticholinergic, antispasmodic muscle relaxer that blocks nerve impulses in the parasympathetic nerve endings, ultimately impeding muscle contractions and spasms in the bladder. While this preparation tends to be less effective than Ditropan, it is also less likely to produce side effects. It too, however, must be monitored for reactions, especially drowsiness, rapid heartbeat, and constipation. (Patients are sometimes warned not to take Pro-Banthine with large doses of antacids or vitamin C, both of which may decrease its effectiveness.)

Finally, Tofranil (imipramine) is sometimes used to treat incontinence by quieting the mechanism that opens the bladder. Since this drug has mood-enhancing effects as well, it can be used in a secondary capacity to combat depression. Several other drugs from various pharmacopoeic families are prescribed for bladder difficulties as well, though most perform functions similar to the medications profiled above.

Catheterization

If medication fails to control bladder problems adequately, the next step is catheterization. This ancient process—there is some evidence that it was practiced by the ancient Egyptians—tends to inspire dread in patients when first recommended, though in fact thousands of MS patients over the years have used catheters and have remained fully capable of normal, productive lives. Proper use, in essence, is a matter of education, psychological adjustment, and common sense.

Two types of catheters are worn: *intermittent* and *indwelling*. An intermittent catheter is employed on an as-needed, self-administered basis whenever the urge to urinate arises. It is attached, used, then removed. An indwelling catheter, is inserted into the penis or urethral opening by a medical professional and remains in place on a permanent or semipermanent basis.

Intermittent catheterization is by far the most preferred of the two methods—indwelling catheters are usually worn only by patients who are physically unable, or psychologically unwilling, to self-administer intermittent catheterization. Even when persons cannot or will not self-catheterize, however, the problem can be circumvented by having a family member or home health aide do the job. Let's have a closer look at how intermittent catheterization works.

Intermittent Catheterization

The intermittent catheter is a safe, effective, and, as one patient called it, "blessedly handy gizmo." Its use is easily learned in a session or two from a medical professional. Provided that privacy is available, it can be used anywhere and at any time by anyone with the need.

The catheter itself is a thin plastic or rubber tube that looks something like a long straw with a plastic bag attached to it, and which works more or less on the same principle as a siphon. When not in use it can be transported in a purse, knapsack, briefcase, or even, if necessary, in a large coat or jacket pocket.

Before it is inserted, the catheter tube is first washed and lubricated, then it is carefully threaded into the penis or urethra, usually while the patient is in a sitting or squatting position. Once in place the tube is pushed slowly and carefully up into the bladder. When the tube is correctly positioned, gravity does the rest, causing the urine to flow down the tube and into the receptacle bag. After the bladder is fully emptied, the catheter is removed, washed in warm, soapy water, and returned to its carrying case till the need arises again, usually within 4 to 6 hours.

Learning to use a catheter can be a frustrating and at times harrowing task, not so much because it is a difficult procedure to master—it is, in fact, fairly easy—but because of the psychic demands it places on patients. Catheter users are, after all, being asked to insert a cold, alien plastic or rubber tube device directly into their bodies, specifically into the most private and psychologically sensitive part of their anatomies. This prospect can be frightening, especially for persons who view the catheter as painful and unhygienic. Couple this with the fact that for some patients catheter use is tantamount to an admission that they have lost control over their basic body functions, and hence, by inference, over other important elements of their lives as well, and the agenda is a loaded one from the start.

But while such fears are common, they tend to be short-lived. Patients soon come to realize how valuable this device really is for helping them establish a normal way of life, and for liberating them from the humiliation of incontinence. Several MS patients speak on the subject:

Lester G.: After a couple of years I started to lose it down there and started pissing in my pants. I tried wearing those padded underwear things but couldn't stand walking around smelling like an outhouse and feeling wet. The medications didn't do much—didn't do *enough*, I should say—so when my doc suggested a catheter I agreed. Before I got to the hospital to learn to use the thing I didn't think much about it. As soon

as I got there though and took one look at the damned thing I
freaked. "That—inside of me!" I thought to myself, and
wanted to run out of there. "No way!" The nurses who showed
me how to use it were okay, but I couldn't go through with it.
I told them I wanted to go home and think about it for a while
before I agreed. Which I did. I did that. It wasn't till another
fourteen months later, when I started going crazy with the
pissing again—it had gotten better for a while, then
worse—that I finally started to use it. Like a lot of the persons
I've talked to since then, I right away saw how easy it is to get
on once you get the knack of it. It's a relief to be able to get
that damned urine out of your body when you want to, instead
of running up to the bathroom every five minutes. It's a
necessary evil, a catheter. Not an evil exactly—a necessary
burden that makes life easier.

Maurine C.: The hardest thing for me was thinking that
other people smelled me. That I stunk. Smelled. That my
catheter smelled. I know that's not very rational. It shows you
the kind of crazy fears you can have. I wash the tube very
carefully before and after, of course. My husband has come to
take it for granted. I don't use it so much now as I did a
couple of years ago. My friends don't care. The ones who are
going to be supportive of you will be that way no matter what
the MS does to you. The ones who are put off by the fact that
you have handicaps are the ones who will fall away early in the
game. MS separates the real friends from the false friends,
that's one thing I learned. I figured with the catheter it would
be the same way. I was right. Some people at work I could tell
were put off right away, especially when they'd walk into the
bathroom and know what I was doing in the stall. Nobody said
anything, but I knew they disapproved. Most of all, *I myself* got
used to it. You get so it just becomes part of your life. I'd hate
to think what I would do now without it.

In certain cases, either because patients have an aversion to
touching their private parts or because motor disabilities make
self-insertion impossible, catheterization can be performed by an-

other person. All that is needed is a willing helper. A patient's spouse can be taught to do the job, a family member, a close friend, or even a professional home aide. Whatever the case, for most helpmates, learning to catheterize another person is relatively simple, and a majority of people get the knack after a few days' practice. If faced with a choice between wearing an indwelling catheter or having intermittent catheterization performed by another person, patients opt for the latter option in almost every case.

Some helps and hints on intermittent catheterization:

• It is good practice to urinate immediately before inserting a catheter.

• When using an intermittent catheter, make sure all urine is thoroughly voided at each session. Patients should never have more than 16 ounces (500 cc) in their bladder at any time.

• Men usually have more need to lubricate catheter tips than women. For both, avoiding Vaseline and similar greasy substances is suggested. Water-soluble gel does the job better, and is less messy. Ask a pharmacist to recommend a good brand. Some people find vaginal lubricating gel a best bet.

• Immediately before having sex, patients are advised to use the catheter to empty their bladders thoroughly. This eliminates leaking and the chance of accidents.

• Have more than one catheter available at all times. Place it in your car, in your school locker, your purse, in a desk, in a drawer at work, wherever. You never know.

• When inserting a catheter, some women find that a small mirror held at the proper reflecting angle improves ease of insertion. A high-wattage light or flashlight improves visibility even more.

• During the first few weeks of catheterization, patients are advised to record the following information in a journal or notebook: the times of day the catheter is used; the amount of urine passed at each voiding; the amount and type of liquids drunk during the day (i.e., 10 ounces of coffee for breakfast, 5 ounces of water at lunch, 7 ounces of tea in the afternoon, etc.); the reasons for urinating each time (i.e., pain, urge, scheduled time, etc.). After several weeks of recording this data, patients will have a map, so to speak, of their voiding patterns which they can use to devise a daily catheterization routine. Once this schedule is established it should be adhered to faithfully. Don't skip, delay, or postpone. A single missed catheter session can invite bladder distension, dribbling, and urinary infection.

• If patients experience sudden spasms in the legs while inserting a catheter tube, this is not necessarily cause for alarm. Stop pushing, relax, wait several moments, then try again. Usually the spasms will pass. Men who suffer an enlarged prostate should consult their physician before using a catheter.

• If for any reason patients have ongoing difficulty inserting the catheter—for men an enlarged prostate can cause trouble—they should go immediately to their physician's office or the emergency room of a local hospital, and have themselves professionally catheterized. Do *not* allow the urine to build up in the bladder. Even if much of the fluid leaks out on its own, the rest will remain trapped and can quickly cause infection.

• Know the signs of urinary infection and watch for them. Typical indications include fever, mucus or blood in the urine, unusually intense urgency or frequency, painful or burning urination, lower back or lower abdominal pain, dark or foul-smelling urinations, and a sudden increase in the amount of residual urine. If one or several of these symptoms occur, consult a physician immediately.

• Persons new to the intermittent catheter are encouraged to discuss their questions with MS patients who have used the device. Just hearing a few well-chosen words of explanation and support is sometimes all that is needed to help patients break through fear and resistance. Experience counts.

The Indwelling Catheter

In certain cases, especially when patients are unable to self-administer intermittent catheters, an indwelling catheter is the best alternative.

Known as the *Foley catheter,* indwelling devices are similar in construction to intermittent catheters, composed of a long plastic tube that empties into a drainage bag at one end and is inserted into the penis or urethral opening at the other. Unlike intermittent catheters, however, Foleys have an inflating device attached to the insertion end of the tube that expands inside the patient's bladder like a balloon and anchors itself there until the device is removed for cleaning, unplugging, or replacement.

An indwelling catheter is far more difficult to fit than the intermittent kind, and the first time it should be put on under sterile conditions by a qualified medical professional. Caregivers who oversee a permanently catheterized patient can learn the technique and *should* learn it for those moments when the catheter becomes clogged. It is essential to do so, however, under a professional's tutelage.

Once in place, the catheter tube must be cleaned near the insertion site with soap and water at least once a day. The bag, which detaches from the end of the tube, is emptied regularly before it fills to capacity, and should be rinsed with a water and alcohol solution. When replaced, the bag must always hang below the patient's groin to let gravity do its job; special catheter clips and hooks to hold the bag in place for wheelchair or bedbound patients can be purchased from medical-equipment stores.

In contrast to intermittent catheterization, Foley users are encouraged to drink as much fluid as possible, especially acidic fruit juices. These prevent calcium salts from building up in the tube, and they acidify the pH of the urine, discouraging growth of infection-causing bacteria. Cranberry juice, orange juice, grapefruit juice, and Vitamin C supplements are all helpful in this regard.

External Catheters

Another form of the intermittent catheter, once the special domain of men but today adapted for women as well, is the external catheter, a device which is placed over the excretory organ rather than inserted into it. Patients use an external catheter by urinating into it, emptying the bag, and then, depending on the make and model, either throwing it away or washing it for further use.

Available in several styles and shapes, including the popular condom catheter, which encloses the penis in a sheath similar to a birth-control-type condom, this device is affixed to the urethra or penis at one end, and on the other to a bag strapped onto the leg. For women a silicone device is fitted into the vagina and held in place by a special bonding cement.

External catheters can be purchased at most pharmacies and medical-supply houses. They offer an excellent alternative for patients who do not wish to use intermittent insertion-type catheters, or who suffer from infections or abnormalities in the genital areas that make intermittent catheters painful and intrusive.

Choosing this device, however, should be done from a position of knowledge rather than guesswork. Talk it over with a physician or nurse. Learn what choices are available. Investigate. Then discuss the matter further with a pharmacist or salesperson at a medical-supply store. There's no harm in experimenting here, and in trying several varieties. Some patients, for instance, alternate between intermittent catheters and external catheters, according to their needs of the moment.

OT Techniques for Persons with Bladder Difficulties

Perhaps the most important OT technique that patients with urgency, frequency, and dribbling problems need for comfortable daily living is simple "restroom-wisdom." This means that in the morning when patients prepare to leave for the day they make certain that they know in advance exactly where they're going and *where in these places the nearest bathrooms are located.* Some tips along these lines from a patient who lives in New York City:

Ben G.: New York is not a good place to get caught if you have to go to the bathroom. Most of the restaurants don't let you use their bathrooms unless you're a customer, and even then they don't all have them. The bathrooms in office buildings are locked, mostly. What I have done in the past is to compile a list of the free or easily accessible bathrooms in the areas of the city I frequent most, and then carry the list with me. I was surprised to learn how many of these "free zones" there are. There are those in the park and museums. Those in coffeeshops. Gas stations. Bus and train stations. Hotels are a great source, but only if the lobby is large enough to enter and leave without being noticed (don't ask at the desk; they'll probably turn you away if I know New York—just use). Bookstores—Barnes and Noble on Eighteenth Street has a terrific one. Certain office buildings have johns that are unlocked, but you have to know which ones. I've also found it's a good trick to carry a letter from my doctor at all times saying I'm an MS patient. Then, if I get stuck and really have to go to the bathroom and there are no johns in sight, I go into the first store I find, show them the letter, and ask if I can use their bathroom. This trick has failed me only once in the many times I've used it.

Further tips for living with a difficult bladder

• For persons who are forced to get up many times during the night to urinate, bathroom safety is a must. Be sure that a night light is kept on at all times. Wear well-fitting night clothes to avoid the possibility of tripping on hanging folds. Know the route you will take between the bed and bathroom inside out. Rehearse it during the day until it becomes second nature. Remove all the electric cords, loose rugs, jutting pieces of furniture that you might stumble into in the dark. For persons with ambulation problems, grab bars and handles should be installed in the bathroom. All small rugs on the bathroom floor should be removed or replaced with rugs that have nonslip bottom surfaces.

• Another trick for frequent night-time urinators is to keep a hand-held plastic urinal at bedside. Commodes adapted for women's needs as well as men's are now available and can be purchased at any pharmacy or medical-supply store. Persons who experience dribbling during the night can protect their mattresses with rubber undersheet coverings, also available at most pharmacies.

• Specially adapted toilet seats, either raised or low, may be useful to persons with bladder disorders—also toilet armrests. Toilets with a front section that removes or is cut out makes catheterizing simpler. See the OT information on spasticity in this chapter for particulars.

• A technique known as the *Credé maneuver* is used by many MS patients to force excess urine out of a distended bladder. Really just a glorified form of body wisdom, the Credé is practiced while sitting on the commode. Place both hands on the lower abdomen. Relax the stomach, begin to urinate, and simultaneously press the hands inward and downward (or in any direction that works best to force out residual urine). Continue to apply pressure until as much fluid as possible is expelled. Some persons start with their hands in the middle of their stomachs and when the urine begins to flow they "guide" it out with regular, downward stroking motions.

Experiment and see which movements achieve the best results. Some patients push down and in on their lower stomachs. Others make circular motions or apply deep, pressing massage to the entire abdominal surfaces. Don't be afraid to press hard; a little extra pressure is sometimes necessary to get the process going.

• Take advantage of every chance you get during the day to empty your bladder. More, not less, is the rule here. Even when a person feels no special urge, the bladder's diminished ability to recognize the need for urination can be deceiving, and it is best to seize the opportunity. Some people simply make it a habit to urinate every hour or even every half-hour. It's also a good idea to urinate automatically before leaving home in the morning, when coming home at night, after each meal, and whenever the bladder feels swollen and full to the touch.

• Always sit down to urinate. This position is more conducive to coaxing out urine than the standing posture. Some people report that the lower they sit the easier it is to void. Others report that high toilet seats help. Experiment.

• For persons with extreme urinary difficulties, several surgical techniques are available. A cystostomy involves the surgical creation of a hole in the bladder and insertion of a drainage tube. A sphincterotomy surgically enlarges the bladder's sphincter muscle. Generally speaking, these and several other surgical methods tend to be successful—but not always, and not always 100 percent. As with any surgical procedure, even minor ones, pain, a mandatory stay in the hospital, and prolonged recovery time are factors that must be considered carefully, along with doctors' fees and hospital expenses. For further particulars on bladder surgery and its feasibility, consult with a physician.

RELIEF FROM PAIN

Although many patients do not suffer acute pain from MS involvement, some do. A few experience it intensely. "It's as if nails were being hammered into the bottom of my feet," one woman described it. "My face feels like lightning is hitting it sometimes," said another.

Clinical attempts at control must, of course, be keyed to the source of the pain, its form, and to its location in the body. Is the pain acute or chronic? Sudden or gradual? Local or generalized? Permanent or intermittent? Can it be traced to the effects of demyelination and hence to the multiple sclerosis itself? Or does it derive from a secondary cause such as tendon swelling, infection, arthritis, compression fractures of the vertebrae, or even from a side effect of medication? Or several of these? Or none? (In some cases pain occurs that patients automatically assume comes from MS, but which upon examination turns out to be entirely unrelated.)

The first job for the clinician, then—if possible—is to identify and isolate the origin of the pain. Treatment can then follow.

Perhaps the most intense suffering MS patients experience is facial pain—trigeminal neuralgia—though happily, no more than 10 percent of patients complain of this disorder. Like other neuralgias or nerve-induced irritations, facial neuralgia comes in sudden, brief paroxysms, targeting a small section of the nerve roots along the gums or chin, and leaving an aching aftermath in the areas affected. Often these bolts of pain respond to over-the-counter analgesics, and in certain cases a dose of aspirin or acetaminophen is all that is needed to keep the problem under control.

More commonly a stronger medication is required, such as Tegretol (carbamazepine). This anticonvulsant drug has been used to treat epilepsy through the years but is now known to help neuralgic facial pain as well. The problem for most people is that the drug takes several weeks to establish a blood level in a patient's system and cannot be taken on an as-needed basis. Side effects such as fatigue, blurred vision, confusion, and nausea are always a possibility, and patients using it must be carefully monitored. Aplastic anemia has been reported in a tiny percent of Tegretol users as well, but this condition can be avoided by having regular blood counts done for patients who use it regularly.

For many persons, facial neuralgia is a transient problem that appears only during exacerbations. Patients affected in this intermittent way quite understandably may wish to avoid the ongoing side effects that regular use of Tegretol entails. In such cases physicians and patients are obliged to work together to determine how frequent the attacks of neuralgia really are, and how severe. Once a clear picture emerges they can then mutually decide whether the benefits of the drug outweigh its drawbacks.

Other drugs given for pain include Dilantin (phenytoin), and the antidepressant Tofranil (imipramine), both of which work in some cases and not in others. For those suffering from optic neuritis, steroid treatment with Prednisone or Dexamethasone often reduces the swelling in the area around the optic nerve and relieves the problem. Again, trial and error are necessary, and side effects are an ever-present possibility. In instances where pain is induced by spasticity, antispastic drugs such as Lioresal often correct the cramping and hence the cause of the suffering. In other situations cold packs, applied physical-therapy techniques, or orthopedic splints and braces bring relief.

Persons who suffer the pins-and-needles of paresthesia or the skin-surface sensitivities of dysthesia frequently obtain an acceptable degree of relief from over-the-counter medications like aspirin. These conditions tend to come and go according to their own mysterious schedules, and after a while many patients simply learn to live with them, especially if the sensations are more an aggravation than an agony. In those instances where they *are* an agony, Dilantin and Tegretol will usually take the edge off, though they will not always stop the hurting entirely.

When and if pain reaches untenable degrees stronger medications may be used and certain forms of surgery and electric treatment are available. For pain of spastic cramps nerve blocks have sometimes been tried, whereby an anesthetic is injected directly into the nerve along the afflicted area. As with other such techniques, results are mixed and inconclusive, though a number of patients claim partial or even full relief from this method. In rare instances the nerves leading to the afflicted areas will be surgically cut to relieve pain, but again this is a chancy procedure, which comes with some risk and no guarantees of success.

Treatment of pain with a TENS unit (transcutaneous electrical nerve stimulation) involves the electrical stimulation of nerve endings along the skin surfaces. By a not entirely understood process, the tiny electrical shocks transmitted through the skin seem to block or divert nerve-originated pain and bring some amount of relief. Statistically speaking, more than 60 percent of general users report some degree of improvement, usually temporary, occasionally long term. Portable TENS units can be purchased for home use, though at a high price, and it is recommended that interested parties test these mechanisms on a thorough basis before making such a costly investment.

COMBATING FATIGUE

Perhaps the most common of all MS symptoms is fatigue. It seems to go along with the MS territory, slowing patients down both physically and psychologically, and proving especially problematic during the weeks and months after a serious flareup.

What can be done to relieve this enervating and seemingly omnipresent condition? Pharmacologically speaking, the choices are limited. Perhaps the only medication doctors have had any success with so far is Symmetrel (amantadine), a drug ordinarily prescribed for the treatment of Parkinson's disease and Asian flu. The reasons why Symmetrel helps MS are not yet understood, for though it appears to promote the release of the neurotransmitter dopamine from the basal ganglia areas of the brain, theoretically this mechanism of action alone should not produce any particular ameliorating effect on MS-related fatigue.

And yet it seems to do just that, and certainly few persons will object. Although there are no assurances here, physicians have found that patients who take this preparation often show a measurable if not dramatic lifting of their pep and energy level, and hence on their general outlook on life. As a bonus, moreover, Symmetrel often improves MS tremor, just as in Parkinson's disease, and is sometimes prescribed specifically for this purpose.

Symmetrel's side effects tend to be minor. Jitteriness and dryness of mouth are both common. Blurred vision can occur and may pose a special difficulty for patients who are already suffering from optic neuritis or glaucoma. If any of these are a problem patients are advised to inform their physicians before taking the drug. Other side effects include constipation, dizziness (especially when standing up suddenly), and a harmless but unsightly skin condition known as *livedo reticularis,* which produces purplish blotches on the thighs or forearms, and which occasionally remains after the medication has been discontinued.

Aside from Symmetrel there are few other medicinal choices in the battle against fatigue. Some doctors report limited success with Cylert (pemoline), a central nervous stimulant used to treat concentration and attention deficits in hyperactive children. Antidepressants may be given, as depression produces a lassitude that is emotional as well as physical in origin. Vitamins such as those in brewer's yeast, Vitamin A, C, E, and the B complex are sometimes touted as energy producers, though these claims remain clinically unproven. Likewise, manganese, zinc, and potassium gluconate supplements, vitamin B_{12} injections, and various megavitamin regimes are used.

Coffee and caffeine drinks are also recommended for tiredness, but these substances do not "give" the body energy, as is commonly believed, they simply stimulate certain organs to produce more of it. Once this effort is expended, an energy deficit is produced, which is often equal and opposite to the energy surge formerly experienced—hence the afternoon "down" complained of by many heavy coffee and soda drinkers and, on a greater scale, by drug-stimulant users. In this sense caffeine and other drugs give with one hand and take back with the other.

In all, the chemical choices for tiredness and fatigue are limited. This means that if fatigue is to be confronted at all it must be done in other ways, specifically by the conservation of energy and by the pacing of one's daily activities. Here a number of things can be done to reduce unnecessary stress and exertions during the course of a day, and the wise patient will incorporate them into his or her lifestyle. In various chapters methods for reducing stress and minimizing exertion (see Chapter 4) are already explained. To supplement this information the following helps and hints can be added:

• Get organized. Old hat, perhaps, but vital to energy conservation. Know where your possessions are—don't waste valuable stores of energy searching for them. Label things. Keep them in plain view. Be systematic. Plan ahead for meals, trips, daily chores. When a sizable job presents itself, don't tackle the whole thing at once. Break the task up into increments, and do a little at a time. "Step by step," goes the saying, "takes one a long way."

• Have the most commonly used household and personal items within easy reach. Remember, MS persons are already starting out with diminished stamina; every time they are forced to stand up and cross the room to retrieve an object that could as easily be kept within reach, unnecessary effort is expended. So keep commonly used items on nearby shelves and tables. Hang the most frequently worn pieces of clothing in an accessible part of the closet. Position kitchen items at shoulder height to avoid bending down. Shelves mounted on cabinet doors eliminate long reaches. Heavy appliances, shop tools, or electronic devices should be kept on a table or counter rather than down below, where they have to be retrieved each time they are used.

• Arrange frequently used chairs, couches, and articles of furniture in locations that are accessible to the centers of activity in a house. Persons who suffer from urinary frequency or nocturia can locate their sleeping quarters near a bathroom to save steps. Better yet, keep a portable commode at the bedside, or anywhere in the house where much time is spent.

• Take advantage of gadgets and mechanical aids. Shelves that pull out or fold down save reaching. So do rotating shelves and lazy susans. Place retracting hooks and hangers in handy places. Use a phone that accesses numbers with single memory-storage buttons. Keep heavy household items on a wheeled cart. Use a clicker for the TV and VCR. Electric blankets place less weight on the legs and are ideal for persons with skin soreness or sensitivity in the lower extremities.

• In the kitchen, electric appliances are more efficient than those worked by hand (a single session spent whipping cream the manual way is enough to exhaust the most healthy homemaker). A self-cleaning oven saves scrubbing efforts; a wall-mounted oven makes bending down unnecessary (some people raise their oven units on blocks for better reach).

• When heavy items must be moved don't drag them; transport them on a dolly. An electric typewriter is easier to use than a manual. An electric toothbrush requires less effort than the manual kind. Electric pencil sharpeners are more energy-efficient than the hand-turning variety. Crock-pots and slow cooking devices save labor. So do blenders and food processors. Intercoms positioned in strategic parts of the home save steps, not to mention vocal cords. For persons in wheelchairs, adequate roll-in spaces beneath counters and under tables are mandatory.

• Keep things in good repair. Household items that don't work properly are energy wasters. If the drawers in a bureau stick and require more effort to open than they are worth, coat the sides with wax or silicone lubricant. Do the same with frequently used windows and doors. Slippery steps can be a hazard—rubber treads or rug coverings will improve traction. A banister installed along a steep staircase is a must when ambulation is a problem (some people place banisters on both sides of the staircase for double security). Wheelchair ramps save effort on steps, both for caregivers and patients. People with vision problems appreciate window glass that sparkles. Patients with vision problems are also advised to use high-wattage light bulbs and position the lamps in their homes for maximum illumination.

• Opt for the most comfortable way to do things. There is no reason, for instance, that a person cannot bring a stool into the kitchen and sit while preparing a meal. Standing uses more energy. The same goes for ironing or working in a shop. Why wash dishes when paper plates and cups can be used? TV dinners and fast foods are easier to prepare than full-course meals; despite their dubious nutritional value, they can be real lifesavers when exhaustion is an issue.

• When taking public transportation, sit, don't stand. Many MS persons find that after walking a short distance a limp or foot drag starts to slow them down. The remedy is to listen to one's body and make frequent rest stops along the way. Take trips, both the long and the short kind, in increments. Be imaginative. If walking to the park with a child, for example, make a game out of stopping at every block or intersection and singing a song, resting for a moment, then continuing on. In many instances, a cane can serve as an extra "leg" and is a real energy saver. Although some patients pale at this thought, when they realize how quickly they and their cane blend into the anonymous landscape, and how helpful it is, it becomes apparent that its benefits outweigh its drawbacks. When journeying to an airport or train station, request a wheelchair and save the energy needed for the rest of the trip. Almost all public transportation centers now provide wheelchairs gratis for persons with disabilities.

• Brick or concrete floors are hard on aching backs and joints, and are dangerous in case of a fall. If it can be afforded, soft carpeting makes easier, safer walking, though persons in a wheelchair may find wood or linoleum preferable. Small scatter rugs already on the floor should be firmly anchored with carpet tacks or Velcro strips. In households with wheelchair patients furniture should be raised or lowered to suit the patients' needs, and all room-to-room routes should be kept clear and accessible for wheelchairs.

• Make home entrances and exits access-easy. For wheelchair patients, entranceways should be smoothly paved and stripped of bumpy impediments. All defects in concrete, stairs, bricks, et al., should be repaired. Good illumination outside the home or apartment is a must, and if possible the garage should be well lighted for safe nighttime coming and going. For wheelchair patients who live in apartments, adequate light is necessary in the hallways, and all dangerous carpeting in the halls should be repaired or replaced.

• When shopping, take a wheeled shopping cart along. Better yet, have the groceries delivered. Patients should not hesitate to ask family members to carry bags that are too heavy or that compromise posture and trigger muscular spasms. Sneakers or running shoes make walking on hard surfaces comfortable (women should *always* avoid heels), though for persons who slip in and out of shoes frequently loafers may be the easier route. Patients who sit for long periods at a desk, table, or counter can save the effort of standing up by placing casters on the chair and wheeling it to their destinations.

All small fixes, perhaps. But when added up these little energy savers amount to big energy savers, and can make a real difference in a patient's level of energy at the end of a day.

HELP FOR AMBULATION

Since many of the gait, balance, and coordination problems of multiple sclerosis are related to spasticity, the medical treatments used for spastic disorders help persons walk better as well. After the regular selection of antispasticity medications have been matched to the person's needs and tolerance level, physical therapy will also be appropriate.

Examples of PT techniques used to help regain walking strength and balance are numerous and are prescribed according to a patient's individual needs and disabilities. In general, a physical therapist will want to determine which muscles are weak, what muscle power and control still remains, and then bring these disparities into balance.

If a person is having difficulties climbing stairs, for example, it may be determined that the difficulty is due to weakness and inflexibility in the leg or ankle muscles. A PT will then select certain muscle sets to stretch out and strengthen with exercise and manipulation.

For balance and walking, posture is a central issue. Two goals are important: one, to prevent patients' posture from worsening, and two, to improve their present posture. Patients may be asked to stand in front of a mirror to study, then self-align, their position. They are told to imagine a plumb line dropping down from the nose to the navel to the knees and feet. Checks are made against tilting, leaning forward, protruding hips, and too much bending at the knees. Once standing posture is corrected, the same modifications will be applied to walking positions.

When patients walk on their own they are helped to become aware of their positions in space and to remain symmetrical in all forward movements, not to tilt, not to sway or tip. Balance issues are addressed. Patients are asked to walk a straight line with a book balanced on the head. They are told to walk the line heel to toe, then perform the same maneuver backward. They may perform braiding movements, balancing on one leg as they walk, then shifting weight to the other, then back again. Base of support and leg spread will be checked, and the width or narrowness of stance corrected.

One mistake frequently made by patients undergoing ambulation rehabilitation is to invent ad hoc exercise programs for themselves that favor muscle groups which are already strong and to neglect those that are weak and in need of work. This lopsided approach causes weak muscles to become weaker and strong muscles to overdevelop. An imbalance results, with leg or trunk muscles working very hard and others working so little that gait is confused and walking coordination thrown out of sync. This condition sets patients up for faulty posture, poor balance, and undue weight distribution, which in turn can trigger spastic reactions.

Physical therapists, moreover, are not only concerned with helping patients walk successfully from point A to point B. They are anxious that bad walking habits be avoided and that a degree of functional independence be returned. Strengthening exercises are thus provided, along with body-awareness techniques, self-righting postural methods, and pacing techniques, whereby patients are taught to walk short distances and then increase these spans as skills develop. The essential point is that ambulation problems *can* be improved, but that in many cases this will happen only when patients are guided through a course of intense corrective therapy.

Finally, as an added aid for walking, orthopedic aids such as walkers, canes, braces, splints, and other tailor-made assistive devices may be recommended, matched to a person's requirements.

AMBULATION AIDS

MS persons with moderate to severe progressive disease often find that in the middle or later stages of their disease, walking becomes increasingly problematic, and they are forced to depend on ambulatory aids to get around.

Know, however, that whatever the degree of disability that exists, there is some form of walking or transportation device that will help. These items can be purchased directly. Or, if you prefer to try out several varieties before making a decision, they can be obtained from a medical-supply house that specializes in rentals.

Let's have a look at how ambulatory devices work and where to find them. The equipment mentioned in this section is available directly from medical-equipment stores, by mail from health-supply equipment catalogs, or through a hospital physical-therapy unit. The address of supply companies mentioned in parentheses after the items listed below are found in the Appendix. It is, however, highly recommended that before purchasing any of these items patients have at least one consultation with a trained physical or occupational therapist to find out which piece of equipment is best suited to their needs, and that they follow the advice they receive to the letter. Ambulation equipment must be carefully matched to the walking requirements of each patient; a wrongly fitted device can be both inefficient and dangerous (an incorrect-sized cane may cause falls; a poorly fitting brace can raise blisters). So check with a trained medical professional first, and then order only when you are clear on your specific needs.

To begin with, don't underestimate the value of the common cane. This old reliable has kept walkers young and old on their feet for centuries, and modern versions are better than ever. Styles include:

- *Standard cane*—Made of lightweight materials such as aluminum, or heavier materials like wood (for those who prefer something natural in their hands), canes come in all shapes and sizes. Adjustable models are handy for tall or short persons (Abbey, Sammons, Cleo).

- *Low-profile quad cane*—Made of anodized aluminum with a chrome-plated steel base and height adjustments. The handle is offset with a foam grip. Very sleek and easy to carry around (Cleo).

- *Quad forearm crutch*—Comes with an adjustable fitting that fastens over the length of the forearm for added strength and balance. This sturdy item can be adjusted for right- or left-hand use (Abbey).

For persons who are especially unsteady on their feet three- and four-pointed canes are sometimes recommended, though there is some debate as to their preferability over the one-legged variety. "Four-point canes reduce the wobble of Grandfather's cane," Dr. John K. Wolf writes,*

> but the mechanics of this cane are only slightly better than Grandfather's. The weakened hand is still at the wrong end of the long fulcrum. The four little feet do not hold the ground much better than the regular cane. A weak hand and arm at the top cannot move the heavy tip quickly and accurately enough to prevent disaster. Consider also the effect of a four-point cane on a person who has just purchased one in order to remain mobile. As he strides confidently along, the little feet stick out about a foot from his side, taking with them the shinbone of a passing pedestrian, with predictable results.

Why not try one yourself and then judge. Varieties include:

• *Four-legged quad cane*—Comes with four toelike legs capped with rubber ends, and a padded foam hand grip (Abbey). Watch out for the cheaper varieties; the rubber end tips wear out quickly.

• *Deluxe lightweight quad cane*—Has special legs that form a wider base than regular four-legged canes. The end tips never need replacing (Abbey).

• *High-base quad cane*—The design of this ingenious device with its raised, spiderlike legs concentrates the weight and provides an improved center of gravity. The problem is that some users find it difficult to transport and ungainly to use. Like most orthopedic equipment, a tradeoff between efficiency of function and ease of use may be required (Abbey).

If ordinary canes do not keep patients well balanced, or if a person's legs are not strong enough to bear the body's weight, a walker is the next possible choice. Be sure to get one that is lightweight and can be adjusted to height. Varieties include:

Mastering Multiple Sclerosis: A Guide to Management. Rutland, Vermont, Academy Books, 1987.

- *Rigid walker*—Usually made of aluminum, this support is the basic, all-purpose walker. Its bolted frame allows for readjustment when needed (Abbey).

- *Wheeled walker*—Comes with wheels on two of the four legs. Though this convenience appears handy at first, the wheels tend to wear out quickly when used on concrete, and for some people a wheeled walker can prove unstable. Be sure to get a PT's opinion on this one (Abbey).

- *Folding walker*—The up side here is that the walker can be folded when not in use and stored in a car or closet. The down side is that it weighs more than other walkers, and has a slightly more complex frame system (Abbey).

Add-on items worth purchasing for a walker include: utility pouches that fit across the handles and hold odds and ends; wire basket for packages and household items; platform attachment for supporting the arms and wrists; and a sling seat that transforms the walker into a chair (all available from Abbey).

Yet another ambulatory aid is the lower leg and ankle splint. MS persons with gait problems often suffer from foot dragging, inturned ankles, and ankles that suddenly go weak and collapse without warning. By strapping on an ankle splint before leaving the house one can often alleviate these problems. For persons who are unsteady on their feet but who do not wish to use a walker or a cane, the splint is a viable alternative. It is, however, suggested that patients discuss the matter fully with their doctors and physical therapists before coming to any decisions. Once a patient's needs are identified, the following varieties of splints are available:

- *Ankle splint*—A lightweight plastic ankle brace that fits over the foot, ankle, and lower leg, fastens with a Velcro strap, and provides surprisingly substantial walking support. Comes in rigid, semirigid, or flexible frame (Cleo).

- *Dorsiflexion elastic assist*—Specifically supports foot drop and assists users in ambulatory training (Cleo).

• *Shoe-clasp ankle-foot orthotic*—A spring-type, short leg brace that runs from the foot up the back of the leg, fastening below the knee. The entire unit clips onto the back of the shoe for easy wearing. An interesting alternative (Cleo).

Some other walking supports that may help:

• *Ankle-support laminate roll*—A flannel-lined elastic material that wraps around the ankle to give extra strength (Cleo). Some MS persons find that a tightly wrapped Ace bandage works just as well.

• *Double-strap ankle support*—A slip-on ankle brace with an open heel that provides compression to both the medial and lateral sides of the ankle (Cleo).

• *Athletic knee pad*—This universal piece of athletic equipment gives extra support to the knee and thus to the entire leg. Buy it at any sporting-goods store.

• *Adjustable thigh support*—A flannel-lined foam elastic support that fastens around the thigh with a hook-and-loop enclosure. It is designed to strengthen the entire leg (Cleo).

• *Overlock knee brace*—A felt and elastic enclosure that braces the entire leg (Cleo).

CHOOSING AND USING A WHEELCHAIR

As with any orthopedic equipment, purchasing or renting a wheelchair is a serious matter and must be approached with as large a knowledge base as possible. Wheelchairs are expensive items. Make one false move, choose a model that doesn't fit through the bathroom door or is too low to the ground or puts too much pressure on the pelvic bone, and patients may find themselves out of pocket for the same item twice in the same year. Third-party payers, moreover, may or may not cover the high cost of a wheelchair the first time around. On the second time, the chances are almost nonexistent. Choosing carefully, preferably with the advice of a physical or occupational therapist, is thus the recommended way to go in this area and can save both pocketbook and health.

"When Mrs. Jones comes in to be fitted out for a chair," Mary Nishimoto, Assistant Director of Physical Therapy Department at Helen Hayes Hospital in Haverstraw, New York, tells us, "the first thing we do is find out whether she actually needs the chair. And we want to know in what capacity she'll be using it. Is it just to get from her home to the doctor's office and back once a week? Will it sit folded up in her closet the rest of the time? Or will she be using the chair for everything she does from the moment she wakes up to the moment until she goes to bed at night? This is vital information. It tells me whether she needs a simple transport chair without the frills or a chair that is more permanent and functional."

When a permanent chair is required, the PT must proceed carefully to the next stage. "The first thing I want to do now is measure Mrs. Jones," says Mary Nishimoto, "to find out how wide she is, how deep her sitting depth is, how long her legs and back are. Will the chair require removable armrests for transfers? Will she need to get in and out often during the day? Should the chair width be standard—eighteen inches wide—or narrow—sixteen inches? Or should it go out to a maximum twenty-four inches? I also have to determine how much strength and mobility Mrs. Jones has in her hands. Perhaps she only has use of one hand, or neither, or one arm and a single leg. In such cases she'll need a specially made chair, and she'll have to be taught how to use it. She may even need a breath-controlled chair or a chin-controlled chair if her arms and legs are immobilized. For persons with one working extremity a power chair or scooter may be the best bet. Or it may not—it depends on their situation."

Once a client's needs are ascertained and their specifications checked, there are other important issues that must be determined. "If Mrs. Jones has both arms available for propelling the chair I'll want to know if her chair is to lean back and recline or remain straight up. And what kind of cushion is best here? This is a complex question for MS patients who are sometimes forced to sit in the most difficult, compromising positions. In these cases the chair has to be matched to the person's postural disabilities, hopefully in a way that has some corrective use in helping the person sit in a more proper way. We always have to worry about pressure sores, especially with clients who are sitting balanced on a couple of bones all day long. We have to make sure the cushion is just right for these folks. It might be a foam cushion, air cushion, gel cushion, or a combination cushion. We have pressure gauges that are inserted between the person's bottom and the cushion to determine how much pressure is there. We know that if the pressure is high, Mrs. Jones is at risk for sores. So we'll change the cushion and lower the risk."

Important too is knowing where the chair will be used. "I'll want to know something about where Mrs. Jones lives. Will the chair fit in her home? How wide are the doorways and entranceways into her house? Especially the bathroom door? What are the floors made of? Is there easy wheeling access to all parts of the house? What about stairs? Will the chair need a special adaptive device to make the climb?" Transportation is an important issue too. "If Mrs. Jones is going to be driven or if she does a lot of driving herself, the chair must be set at a certain height so she can transfer easily from the chair to the car and back again. And will she need a device that lifts her chair mechanically to the roof of the car for storage? Might she need a van to transport the chair in? If the chair folds, will it fit into the trunk of her car?"

How will patients know if a wheelchair is right for them? Two ways. First, if a chair does not fit properly their backs and buttocks will tell them. Second, within the first few days or weeks of use patients will experience unusual physical problems: backaches, neck pains, pressure sores. Or, in another scenario, a patient will find that his or her chair is adequately comfortable but mechanical and logistic difficulties make it useless—difficulties such as not being able to reach the wheel, or a seat that is so low the patient cannot stand up.

Then there are the bells and whistles. "Some patients, especially young ones," Mary Nishimoto tells us, "like power wheelchairs—chairs you can run with an electronic central control unit.

These devices are very versatile. Not only do the seat and back give a lot of support but there is more surface area in general, and power chairs accept more styles of supportive back rests. Since some of our clients have trouble sitting up straight this can be a real asset; they literally need a chair back that hugs them.

"If clients are careful about picking the right chair they will find one that is adaptable to their problems and that has a lot of the work done for them by these controls, such as the main joystick. Say, for example, that a person has bad ataxia. If this person's arms are flying all around they can't control the joystick. So there are gadgets on the power chair that allow them to switch over to electronic control of the chair with their chins or breath. They can also change the joystick from the right-hand side to the left if the range of motion of an extremity starts to deteriorate. Some chairs will even sit you up or stand you up when you tell them too. Others have a computer attached to them by which severely disabled patients can control the room temperature, turn on the lights and TV and stereo, make a phone call, all while they're sitting in their chair. The possibilities today, with exploding medical technology, are remarkable and endless."

TREATING TREMORS

Tremors are common among MS patients, though their range and intensity vary markedly. Some persons with ataxia will present with wide excursions of movement in the arms and hands, and will be unable to perform the most simple manual task such as buttoning a shirt or guiding a spoon to the mouth. These tremors are not in the majority, fortunately. More often a subtle oscillation of the head or trunk appears and disappears periodically, and often goes unnoticed by others.

When shaking is slight, patients are able to compensate with simple tricks such as keeping their arms close to their bodies when making arm movements or using adaptive devices to accomplish difficult manual tasks. In instances where tremors are exacerbated by emotional agitation, the sedative effect of antihistamine drugs such as Atarax (hydroxyzine) will relax the person and thus the shaking. In still other cases Inderal (propranolol), a blood pressure and angina medication, produces improvement and is most effective in cerebellar tremors that originate in the basal ganglia part of the brain.

As mentioned above, Symmetrel is sometimes prescribed for shaking and has the added effect in some patients of relieving exhaustion. When a tremor is related to spasticity, antispasticity drugs such as Lioresal may slow it down enough to restore functionality to the affected parts. Finally, there is some evidence that Isoniazid, one of the three major drugs used for treating tuberculosis, has a tremor-dampening effect, especially for a severe tremor. Since this drug tends to produce liver toxicity in the large doses necessary for tremor control, however, and since it is a relative newcomer to the MS pharmaceutical canon, its use is controversial and should be considered only in extreme cases, and then only when accompanied by regular liver-function studies. Patients are advised to discuss this matter with their physicians. Overall, it should be added, pharmacologic treatment of MS tremor is disappointing, and as yet no single drug achieves anything approaching total success.

Other methods for controlling tremor include:

• *Weights*—A compensatory technique in which weights are attached to shaking limbs, especially ankles or wrists. This technique is designed to involve peripheral muscle groups in movement efforts and thus add extra muscular control to the limbs to keep them from shaking. Similar help can be achieved by using heavy objects for everyday manual tasks such as weighted writing instruments, eating utensils and brushes.

• *Exercise*—Physical therapists often recommend exercises that concentrate on stability, especially of the shoulder, pelvis, hips, and trunk. An exercise known as *patterning* requires patients to repeat certain movements many times with resistance added by the PT as the movements become increasingly automatic. With repeated practice these motion patterns become fixed in the body's muscular memory and, to some extent, reprogram and improve motor skills.

• *Orthopedic equipment*—In cases where control is lost over movement of the head and neck, special braces are fitted that exert an inhibiting "straitjacket" effect on the shaking. Hands and feet may also be immobilized in this way, usually on a temporary basis.

• *Surgery*—In cases of chronic cerebellar tremor a form of surgery known as a *thalamotomy* is performed in which the tremor-generating part of the thalamus gland is destroyed by freezing or cutting. This operation is rare and practiced only in cases where the tremor is extreme and fails to respond to other forms of therapy. Thalamotomies are also used in general surgical practice to remedy harsh and untreatable pain.

ALLEVIATING SPEECH AND SWALLOWING DISORDERS

The type of speech and swallowing disorders developed by MS patients depends on which area of the brain is demyelinated, and, in turn, which parts of the tongue, lips, larynx, vocal cords, and throat are affected. Speech may be slurred, unusually rapid, eccentric in rhythm, weak, or choppy. Swallowing reflexes may be impeded or delayed; sensations in the oral passageways may be severely diminished.

In cases of speech or swallowing disorders—both, happily, are relatively rare among MS sufferers—there is little that can be done from a pharmacologic standpoint, and the brunt of the work will involve management and rehabilitation. Speech language pathologists specialize in swallowing and speech problems, using such techniques as diet modification, special food preparation techniques, mouth and throat exercises, postural modification, and muscle-retraining techniques, all of which at times can prove extremely effective.

If speech or swallowing difficulties occur during the course of the disease, a physician should be consulted for referrals to a licensed speech pathologist.

HELP FOR VISION PROBLEMS

Optic neuritis is a relatively common symptom among MS patients, though it tends to be transient and is often best treated by allowing the flareup to pass on its own. When and if the neuritis becomes severe, and especially if acute loss or distortion of vision occurs, steroid treatment will reduce inflammation in the optic centers and bring the visual faculties into working order.

In some cases, as mentioned earlier, even after the condition has been treated and the inflammation subsides, residual sight deficiencies may linger. Often these problems will self-correct. Occasionally they become permanent, though blindness per se is extremely rare. In many instances, corrective lenses, eye patches, and other ophthalmological aids are available to offset these deficiencies.*

---

*The authors wish to thank Janet Gray and Margaret Knowland, chief nurses at the Multiple Sclerosis Unit at Helen Hayes Hospital in Haverstraw, New York, for their valuable contributions to several sections in this chapter.

6

Exercise

Over the past several decades physical exercise has emerged as a superstar in the development of enduring health. Exercise is now known to confer a wide range of benefits to the human organism, some subtle, some noticeable right away. Circulation is increased and improved. Muscles are made stronger, as are the muscle-ligament connections. The cardiovascular system is strengthened, and increased supplies of cell-building oxygen are transported to tissues throughout the body. Exercise accelerates removal of waste products from the body, stimulates the bowels, reduces blood pressure, cleans the pores of the skin. It is known to elevate the number of high-density lipoproteins in the blood, thus giving exercisers some measure of protection against atherosclerosis and stroke.

The list continues, and there is no doubt that physical exercise, when carried out on a safe, regular daily schedule, is a substantial boon to health. The question that concerns us here, however, is whether exercise is beneficial to MS patients in particular?

The answer is yes—but with several important cautions to consider first.

MS AND EXERCISE: SOME CAVEATS

For many years MS patients were advised *never* to exercise, to remain as calm and stationary as possible at all times, and to let others do the work for them. Too much physical exertion, it was believed, brought on fatigue and perhaps symptom flareups. Continual, ongoing rest was the standard prescription. No exceptions tolerated.

Today the attitude of medical professionals has taken a full 180-degree turn, and most health-care workers now agree that exercise is beneficial for MS, sometimes highly beneficial, but—*but*—that several critical precautions must be taken first if it is to be used in a successful way.

The most important of these precautions is that an MS exerciser must never—*never*—overdo. Following the "stretch it till it hurts, and then some" philosophy is not only counterproductive, it can end up producing results diametrically opposed to good health, straining an already compromised muscular system, increasing pain, causing a person to become overtired, overheated, overstressed.

It is thus urged—and this is the second caution—that before beginning a workout regime MS patients check with a physician or physical therapist. Under normal circumstances, for instance, healthy people with lower-back problems may be told to practice regular regimes of lower-back calisthenics. An MS person, however, may have neurological disturbances in the lower back, and exercising this area could possibly make the symptoms worse. Stretches and twists in other parts of the body may be perfectly okay for such patients. The patient simply must avoid exertions in the problem areas. Many similar examples could be cited.

So check first. In general, the type of exercises that will be recommended for MS persons depends on their prevalent symptoms, the potential for harming certain organs and muscle groups, and a person's energy level and overall state of health. Health-care professionals will have recommendations to make on one or more of the following:

1. The type of exercise best suited to one's needs and stamina level.
2. The type of exercises to avoid, and what body systems not to overstress.
3. How much exertion is recommended during each session.
4. The amount of time to exercise and the physical limits that should be placed on each daily workout session.
5. Referrals to other professionals, such as rehabilitation therapists who can tailor-make exercises to one's specific needs.

Note that scientific methods of "exercise testing" are available to help determine such critical elements as an MS person's maximum exertion rate, oxygen-uptake capacity, heart rate, and so forth. Once established, these guidelines are used to recommend a program based on a patient's tested fitness level, fatigue capacity, and general physical abilities. If patients have questions relating to their exercise limits and wish to have a workout program tailored to their needs, they should discuss the matter with a physical therapist or sports-medicine specialist, a majority of whom are trained in exercise testing.

Finally, a general piece of advice: If patients do get the green light on exercise, they are advised to make haste slowly. Note:

• If you plan to exercise for a half-hour during each session, start with ten-minute sessions and build up to the thirty-minute goal over a period of several weeks. An incremental approach is best.

• Three or four exercise periods a week are probably adequate. Most MS patients find that overexercising produces diminishing returns and tends to be globally tiring, upping an exerciser's chances of injury, falls, and fatigue.

• Work out in a safe environment. Avoid slippery floors, dangling lamp cords, poor lighting, unanchored throw rugs, and so on.

• Warm up at the beginning of each session, then cool down at the end. A rule of thumb: for every half-hour exercise session, spend five minutes warming up and five minutes cooling down. For an hour session, spend ten minutes warming up, ten cooling down.

• Beware of hyperventilation and overheating. Both are harmful to MS patients, and both can bring on symptoms. Exercise to the point of gentle stimulation, *not* to the point of dripping with sweat like a marathon runner.

• Persons with balance problems should exercise within reach of a grab bar or guard rail. Sight- or balance-impaired persons can hold the back of a sturdy chair when exercising. In regard to these and other safety measures, seek the advice of a medical professional.

• If an exercise hurts in any way, STOP DOING IT RIGHT NOW! This is critical. Exercisers should allow their bodies to tell them what is right and what is wrong. Even if a medical professional has given the okay on a certain exercise, when something inside says "uh uh," take note. This is body wisdom speaking. Listen to it.

GO TO IT!

In the pages that follow several systematized exercise programs are provided. Sections are divided into exercises for the ambulatory, for the wheelchair-bound, and (to be done with a caregiver) for MS persons confined to bed.

A few words of advice before beginning:

1. Avoid stressing sore or aching parts of the body. Work out until pleasantly stimulated, but *never* to the point of pain. If unusual pains of any kind occur while exercising, discuss this matter immediately with a doctor or physical therapist before continuing.

2. Wear comfortable, loose-fitting clothing. Avoid clothes that bind or trip. Keep loose cuffs and shirttails tucked in, shoes tightly laced (Velcro fasteners are preferable to shoelaces). Loose sweatshirts and pants are the best clothes for exercising.

3. Take short, frequent rests. If fatigued at any time, stop, then either take a break or pack it in for the day. Then pick up again tomorrow.

4. The number of repetitions specified in the following exercise programs are only suggestions. Use them as guidelines, but remember that nothing is written in stone. If you feel comfortable doing fewer repetitions of a particular exercise—or more—by all means follow your instincts.

5. Some repeat advice: Don't push it. Relax. Take it slow. Remember, workout time is neither a competition nor an endurance contest. Patients are not out to set a record or to beat the clock. Pacing is important. Take your time. Have fun.

6. And a final reiteration: If any of the following exercises cause discomfort, discontinue them immediately. Do not practice any exercise that compromises one's condition or places undue pressure on a sensitive part. Any questions in this area should be discussed with a medical health-care professional.

The following is a light to moderate exercise workout for ambulatory patients.

Exercise Group 1: Warmups

• Lie on your back. Bend your right leg to your chest, hold for a moment (pulling it tight to your chest if there is no discomfort), then back to the floor. Do the same with the left leg, lifting, bending, back to the floor. Alternate between rapid right and left leg lifts for several minutes.

• Lie on your back. Extend your arms up over your head and, parallel to the floor, and stretch. At the same time stretch your hips and legs down in the opposite direction. Imagine that two people are having a tug of war with your spine as the rope. Hold this stretch for 5 seconds, relax, then repeat several times.

• On your back, extend your arms straight out to the sides (so that your body forms a cross) and stretch them vigorously. Then raise your arms up and over your chest, and stretch upward. Then back to your sides for another stretch. Repeat this sequence several times.

- Do 10 sit-ups, pacing yourself. Don't strain. Go slowly. If you have the go-ahead from a physical therapist on this exercise, do several sets in a row, but never to the point of fatigue or overheating.

- Start on your back, then rise to a sitting position. Touch your left hand to your right foot, stretch for a moment, then reverse, touching your right hand to your left foot. Alternate several times.

- Assume a comfortable standing position with your feet under your shoulders and your arms at your sides. Bend at the waist and let your arms dangle freely downward, reaching out to touch your toes (don't strain or push). Take deep breaths and relax. Remain in this position for several minutes, then slowly straighten up. Repeat several times.

- Rapidly raise and lower yourself on your toes 10 times. Do several repetitions.

- Lift your right leg at the knee (holding a grab bar or back of a chair to steady yourself if necessary). Pull the leg to your chest with one hand, return to the floor, and repeat with the left leg. Alternate 10 times in rapid sequence. Then march in place briskly for 30 seconds.

- From a standing position, lift your left leg and rotate the left ankle clockwise for several turns, then counterclockwise. Repeat with the right leg. Continue until your ankle joints feel comfortably tired.

- Place the palms of both hands against a wall. Keeping your hands in place, step back several feet, allowing your hands to support most of your body weight. Lift your left heel, keeping the ball of the left foot on the floor and the right knee straight, with the body leaning forward. Get a good stretch on the right calf.

Now reverse: lift the right heel, stretching the left calf. Repeat 10 times for each leg. Be careful of this exercise if balance or standing orientation is a problem.

• Extend your arms in front of you. Rotate the left hand at the wrist clockwise, then counterclockwise, for 10 turns, then do the same with the right. Repeat several times.

• With arms extended in front of you, shake your hands rag-doll fashion for several minutes, then rotate your right arm in wide sweeping circles clockwise, then counterclockwise. Do the same with the left arm. Alternate arms. If any unusual pain is felt in the joints or muscles, stop immediately.

• Walk in place briskly for several minutes. If you wish to increase the aerobic value of this exercise clap your hands over your head as you walk, then bring them down and slap your thighs, then clap over your head again, down to the sides, etc., as if doing a form of jumping jacks. Proceed with caution if you have leg or back problems. Don't go too fast.

Exercise Group 2: For the Back, Trunk, and Limbs

• Lie face down on the floor. Pushing up with the arms, lift your head, shoulders, and upper trunk off the floor (the hips, thighs, and legs remain flat). Support yourself in this sphinxlike position, giving a comfortable stretch and arch to the spine. Hold for 20 seconds, relax, then repeat 2 more times.

• Lie on your stomach with your head on the floor and your hands clasped under your chin. Slowly raise your left leg, keeping your pelvis and right leg flat on the floor. Keep the leg suspended for 5 seconds, then slowly bring it down. Repeat the same movement with the right leg. Perform several sets in a row.

• Lie on your back, knees bent. Tuck the knees to your chest, then slowly raise both legs until they form a right angle to the floor. Your hands should be under your buttocks for support, lower back flat on the floor, knees and feet touching, legs straight, toes pointed. Hold for several moments, then lower. Repeat several times.

• Lie on your back. Press the pelvis and small of your back firmly down to the floor for 5 seconds, tightening your buttocks and abdominal muscles as you push. Relax and release. Repeat 10 times. When practicing this exercise, your stomach should be sucked in. The more downward local pressure you apply in the small of the back the better. This exercise is especially good for lower back spasms.

• Lie on your back. Pull your right knee smartly to your chest and hug it, keeping your left leg on the floor, slightly flexed. Lift your head toward the hugged knee. Hold it there for 10 seconds, then lie back onto the floor. Repeat with the other leg.

• Lie on your back with the small of the back pressed to the floor. Grasp both knees and hug them to the chest, then release. Repeat 10 times.

• Sit on the floor with the legs extended straight out in front. Clasp your hands behind your back. Keeping the arms straight, squeeze your shoulder blades together, trying to make your elbows touch. Hold this position for 5 seconds, then release. Repeat several times.

• Stand up. Position yourself with your back against a wall, feet about four inches from the base. Tighten your stomach and press the lower and middle back against the wall, bending the knees slightly. Keep your chin tucked in to your chest. Repeat several times.

• From a standing position, clasp your hands behind your back and slowly bend over, keeping your arms straight and giving a good stretch to the shoulders, back, hips, and upper legs. Hold this position for 10 seconds, then slowly rise up. Repeat several times. You can perform this same exercise while sitting cross-legged or kneeling as well.

• Stand with your back against a wall. Bending your knees and pressing your spine against the wall, slowly slide to a sitting position—back straight, legs bent as if seated in a chair. Hold this position for 5 seconds, then slide up to a standing posture. With a bit of practice you should be able to remain in the back-against-the-wall seated position for 20 or 30 seconds at a time. It is an excellent exercise for increasing back strength and flexibility. If you have balance problems, consult with a health-care professional first before trying this one.

• From a standing position, extend your arms over your head with palms flat and facing up. Stretch vigorously upward; reach for the sky.

Maintain this stretched posture for approximately 20 seconds, then lower your arms to the side until they are parallel to the ground (your body is now forming a cross). Hold for 15 to 20 seconds, giving a good stretch to the elbows, wrists, and forearms.

Finally, drop your arms to your sides. With palms flat and as nearly parallel to the floor as possible, push vigorously downward, holding this stretch for approximately 20 seconds.

Continue to alternate between the upward, side, and downward stretches, holding each for 5 to 10 seconds. Do as many sets as feel comfortable.

• In a standing position, rotate your hips clockwise several times, then counterclockwise.

Exercise Group 3: For the Head, Face, Neck, and Arms

• Clasp your arms behind your back, if possible gripping your right elbow with the left hand and left elbow with the right hand (don't force it). Rotate your neck for several minutes, first in one direction, then the other. You should feel a wonderful stretch in your neck, shoulders, and upper arms.

• Shrug your shoulders briskly 10 times. Take a deep breath. Then alternate shoulder shrugs, raising your left shoulder, then your right, left, right, etc., in rapid succession. Do 10 shrugs with each shoulder, and more if it feels comfortable.

• Rotate your head clockwise several times, then counterclockwise. Get a deep stretch in the neck in both directions.

• Jut your chin and jaw as far out as they will go, then pull them back in as far as they will go. Perform 10 repetitions.

• Bend your head to the right and try to touch your right ear to your right shoulder. You won't succeed, but no matter (don't force it). Make the same movement to the left shoulder. Alternate from right side to left side 10 times.

• Crane your neck straight up and away from your shoulders for several seconds, then push your head down like a turtle into your shoulders. Alternate these expanding-contracting movements several times.

• Open your mouth as wide as it will go, close it, open it, close it, etc. Repeat a number of times in succession. Next, tighten and loosen the muscles in your nose, mouth, forehead, eyes, and scalp. Stick out your tongue and hold it extended for several seconds. Wrinkle your brow several times, and puff out your cheeks.

• Scrunch your face, tightening the muscles in the forehead, cheeks, mouth, ears, and chin. Hold for several beats, then relax. Scrunch again. Repeat this exercise several times, giving as many of the muscles in your face a workout as possible. When finished, rub your face with the palms of your hands vigorously for 10 seconds. Note: The face is often neglected in exercise systems; it has many significant muscles that require stimulation and stretching.

Exercise Group 4: Cooling Down

The session is coming to a close. So slow down, calm down, bring down your exertion rate before you call it quits. Cooling off allows the heart rate to decrease gradually, the muscles to detense, the metabolism to readjust. Here are some suggestions:

• Shrug your shoulders slowly and rhythmically for 30 seconds.

• Turn your head gently from side to side.

• Reach and stretch your right arm, then your left arm diagonally across your body. Alternate at a slow, steady pace.

• Sit on the floor and slowly bend over, reaching out for your toes. Don't strain. Remain in this bent-over position for several minutes, easing your shoulders forward and extending your hands.

• Sit on the floor with your legs spread in front of you in a wide V. Have someone stand behind you and gently push your upper torso to the floor, giving a good stretch to your lower back, hamstrings, and hips. Your helper should be extremely gentle, pushing with easy, steady pressure. After several minutes rise up slowly and carefully. You should feel relaxed now and wonderfully stretched out.

• Rub your face briskly. Massage and gently pat your scalp and the back of your head. Rub your ears, temples, and neck. Stretch your whole body. Take several deep breaths. Release. Relax. Rest.

The following are vigorous exercises for MS persons who are fit and ambulatory. Use them as a supplement to the exercises above.

• *Yoga*—The ancient Indian system of lifts, stretches, thrusts, and twists is an accessible and effective method of moving the entire body through various range-of-motion positions. Because yoga concentrates on stretching the joints rather than compressing or pounding them (as in jogging and certain calisthenics), this method is ideally suited to improving flexibility and energy level.

A large number of yogic exercises are performed lying down, thus protecting the seeing-impaired or balance-impaired exerciser from trips and falls. Do be careful, however, of the pretzel-type positions you may see in books on the subject. These are for advanced practitioners only, and can cause damage even to seasoned exercisers. Stick with the elementary exercises.

Yoga classes are given in most communities today. Be sure your instructor is certified, and that all exercises are in line with the safety standards set by a doctor or physical therapist. (A number of yoga teachers today, it should be mentioned, have been trained in physical therapy as well and can design a regime of yogic exercises specific to a patient's needs.)

• *Aerobics*—Those who have the go-ahead from their physician to perform aerobics will find these exercises an excellent stimulant for the heart, lungs, and circulation, as well as a satisfactory compromise for runners who no longer have the stamina for prolonged jogging.

Be careful not to overdo. Warm up first, cool down last, and pace yourself throughout. Avoid overheating and getting out of breath. Persons practicing aerobic exercises are urged to do so under the watchful eye of a physical or exercise therapist. Many hospitals and MS groups hold regular aerobic sessions, most of them overseen by professionals. Find out when these sessions meet from your physician or MS chapter.

• *Jogging*—Jogging is hard on the joints. So jog on soft ground or a cinder track whenever possible. Use well-balanced running shoes, making certain the laces are tight. Don't become winded or overheated. At the first sign of dizziness, foot dragging, or balance loss stop immediately. Overall, proceed in this with great caution and only when having first checked with a medical professional.

• *Biking*—Another exercise for the especially fit MS patient. Be careful if motor coordination or balance is a problem: one flying spill is guaranteed to ruin your day.

If you feel nervous at the prospect of biking, a safe and expedient substitute is a home cycling machine. You can pedal these machines several miles a day and never leave the safety of your bedroom. Biking exercisers are affordable, especially the small portable models, and produce most of the health benefits of real biking, but without the risk. They can be purchased at any sporting-goods or exercise-equipment store.

• *Walking*—For most active MS persons, fast (or even slow) walking is a more attractive exercise alternative than jogging, and this for several reasons. Walking is less physically exhausting, safer, and can be done in practically any urban, suburban, or rural environment. Under a worst-case scenario, it can even be done at home around one's dining-room table (don't laugh—one male MS patient who feels insecure about walking on the street keeps fit by strutting up and down his hallway with a cane 20 times in the morning and 20 times at night).

Vigorous walking provides the body with almost as many health benefits as running and at the same time presents fewer hazards to the joints, the heart, and one's sense of motor control. Walking can be a pleasant community event; many MS groups encourage members to take regular strolls as a group or in pairs, thus getting social as well as physical mileage from their exercise sessions.

How far should you walk each day?

It all depends on your condition, stamina, and time. A mile or two is enough for most people. For some, less is better, for some, more. Check with a medical professional. Do be assured, however, that if you walk briskly at least once a day, either assisted or on your own, the results will soon become apparent, both in your fitness level and in your state of mind.

• *Swimming*—Swimming has been called the perfect exercise, and with good reason. Water creates a weightless medium, providing a natural source of resistance that brings gentle but firm exercise to every part of the body. Swimming allows the joints to move through their full range of motion and offers a stimulating workout for the cardiovascular system. Water, moreover, is a healing substance in its own right—cool, invigorating, therapeutic. Even a five-minute dip can lift the spirits.

A few cautions, however. Be sure the pool is not too hot. Pools set at 90 degrees or more may cause the kind of flareup produced by a sauna or hot shower. Be careful also of developing muscle spasms while swimming; stay out of the deep end unless a good swimmer is present to assist you.

Avoid staying under water too long, or stressing your lungs. Swim only in places where a lifeguard is on duty. Movement-impaired MS patients can get their swim time by wearing inflatable "floaties" that slip onto the arms and keep swimmers buoyant. Floaties can be purchased at any variety shop or toy store.

Here are some exercise dos and don'ts for ambulatory MS persons:

- DON'T exercise strenuously one day, skip four or five days, then exercise twice as hard on the sixth. Lost exercise cannot be compensated for by periodic exercise binges. Remain faithful to a regular schedule and avoid inconsistency.

- DO always warm up.

- DO always cool down.

- DON'T perform vigorous exercise the moment you wake up in the morning.

- DON'T exercise when you are fatigued or sleepy, or after you have just eaten a heavy meal.

- DON'T exercise for at least seven hours after you have drunk alcohol, especially if you suffer from balance or gait problems.

- DO drink plenty of water before and after every exercise session.

- DON'T eat for at least one hour before you begin exercising.

- DON'T exercise at bedtime if you suffer from sleep disorders. Exercise raises the body temperature and may interfere with sleep.

- DON'T hyperventilate or hold your breath for long periods of time while exercising.

- DON'T work out for long periods of time on a hard surface. A soft rubber mat, a rug, plus a pair of light, well-padded shoes will absorb pounding on your joints and spine.

- DO exercise during the times of day when you have the most energy.

- DO empty your bladder before beginning each exercise session.

- DO wear all braces or orthopedic devices necessary for the support of weakened limbs.

• DO exercise in a well-ventilated, open space free from household objects to bump into or trip over. If you exercise in a park or backyard, be careful: lawns are deceptively bumpy and uneven. Be sure a steadying device of some kind is nearby; that you wear proper shoes; and that you exercise on a flat, friendly, soft (but not too soft) surface.

• DO take frequent rests. Exercise is a therapeutic recreation designed to make you feel better and to improve your overall bodily functioning. The only person you must please in this regard is yourself.

Exercise for the Wheelchair-Bound

Most of the cautions mentioned above apply as well to wheelchair patients. Note also the following:

1. Talk to a health-care professional before starting an exercise program.

2. Meet with a physical therapist or other rehabilitative specialist who can prescribe exercises especially suited to your needs and disabilities.

3. Avoid exercises that stress a vulnerable or disabled part of the body. Consult with a medical professional concerning which kinds of exercises you should *never* do.

4. Warm up at the beginning of each exercise session and cool down at the end. Pace yourself throughout.

5. Avoid overheating and becoming winded.

6. Don't strain; don't push; don't overtire; husband your physical resources. Make haste slowly.

Since patients confined part time or full time to a wheelchair have differing levels of strength, energy, motivation, and disability, the degree of difficulty and the number of repetitions listed here are simply general guidelines. Increase them or decrease them according to your needs.

Note also that patients with severe disabilities may find it difficult or painful to perform certain of the movements explained below. No doubt patients who have lost use of their legs will wish to skip over the leg lifts and concentrate on the upper-torso exercises instead. At the same time—and here you must seek advice from a physician or physical therapist—exercises for poorly functioning parts of the body can in some instances bring about rehabilitative changes and improvement. Perhaps it's worth a try.

Wheelchair-bound patients, moreover, remain in the same posture for long periods of the day, making them prone to the problems that physical inactivity brings—stiffness, poor circulation, sluggish bowels, pressure sores, and an overall feeling of apathy and malaise. It is thus recommended that a daily or every-other-day exercise routine be faithfully adhered to. Don't underestimate the value of small exertions in this department. In many cases even a few minutes of mild daily exercise can overcome many of the troubles that result from immobility.

The following is an exercise program for the wheelchair-bound MS patient.

Exercise Set 1: Warmup

• Sit upright in your chair, back as straight as it will go and head up. Take 4 or 5 deep breaths. Get as comfortable as possible. Relax. Take several more breaths.

• (If possible) lift your right leg off the floor, hold it up for a moment, then return. Lift the left leg, hold, return. Alternate back and forth. If your legs do not work on their own, you can clasp your hands underneath them and lift. Or you can skip this exercise entirely. The same with the next.

• (If possible) place your feet together on the floor and rapidly fan your legs out and in at the knees for 20 seconds. Stop, rest, relax for a moment, then do another repetition of 20 fans. You can move your legs with your hands if necessary.

• Bending at the hip, lean to your right as far as you can comfortably go. Hold for a moment, then return to an upright position. Lean to your left side, hold, return. Do 5 leans to each side.

• Lift your right arm straight over your head, give it a good stretch at the shoulder, then bring it down. Repeat with the left: lift, stretch, return. Alternate between arms at a brisk pace until you feel comfortably tired.

• Extend your right arm to the side parallel to the floor. Give it a good stretch, then return. Do the same with the left arm: extend, stretch, return. Alternate between arms at a brisk pace until you feel comfortably tired.

• Extend both arms straight out in front of you. Rotate the wrists several times in each direction, then move your arms to the sides (parallel to the floor) and rotate the wrists several more times. Return your arms to your lap, rest a moment, then do several more repetitions.

• Lift both arms over your head, stretch for a moment, then return them to the lap. Lift again, stretch, and back to the lap. Do 20 rapid repetitions. Breathe deeply and evenly as you exercise.

• This time extend both arms out to your sides so that they are parallel to the ground. Make a quick stretch at the shoulder joints, then bring the arms back to your chest. Now out again, back again, out, back. Do 20 rapid repetitions.

• Rotate your right arm a full 360 degrees in its socket. Then the left. Perform 5 full rotations with each arm.

• Rotate your head counterclockwise several times, then clockwise. Get a good stretch in the shoulders and the neck.

• Shrug your shoulders 20 times. Rest for a moment. Then lift your left shoulder, drop it, your right shoulder, drop it. Alternate, 10 lifts on each side.

• Jut your chin out as far as it will go, then pull it back in as far as it will go.

- Rub your face briskly 30 times.

Exercise Set 2: For the Legs and Lower Torso

Note: Many MS patients confined to a wheelchair suffer from disabilities in the legs. Certain of the following exercises may be inappropriate. If you have any questions along these lines, consult with a health-care professional.

- Extend your right leg straight out as far as it will go. You may wish to use your hands to assist you in extending the leg. It doesn't matter how far out your leg reaches; whatever distance you attain is good. Stretch your leg vigorously for several moments, bend it at the knee, then place it back on the floor. Repeat with the left leg. Alternate several times.

- Extend your right leg out as far as it will go. Rotate your foot at the ankle 5 times clockwise and 5 times counterclockwise (or as many times as feel comfortable).

- Extend your right leg, point the foot, getting a good ankle stretch, then rotate and return. Repeat with the left leg. Repeat several times.

- Sitting straight in your chair, bend your body as far forward as you can comfortably go, bracing yourself with your feet. Once hunched over, push yourself back with your feet into a sitting position, then rock forward again, then back, then forward, establishing a slow, rhythmic motion. Continue this exercise for several minutes, being sure to get a strong stretch on your feet, ankles, and calves every time.

- Sitting straight in the chair, extend your lower torso in an upward direction, getting a stretch in the abdomen and spine. Hold for several moments, then relax. Alternate several times.

- Sitting straight in the chair, bend your upper torso to the right, hold, then repeat to the left. Alternate several times.

- Sitting straight in the chair and keeping your buttocks firmly based on the seat, rotate your hips 360 degrees in a clockwise motion so that your lower torso receives a full range-of-motion workout. Then rotate counterclockwise several turns. Don't strain.

Exercise Set 3: For Upper Torso, Arms, Neck, and Head

• Start with your hands in your lap. Extend your arms straight out in front, parallel to the floor. Hold this position for 3 or 4 seconds, getting a good stretch in the shoulders and elbows, then return. Repeat 10 times. Next, extend your arms straight out to your sides. Hold and stretch for 3 or 4 seconds. Do 10 repetitions. Reach your arms straight over your head as if making the touchdown sign and stretch. Finally, keeping your arms stiff at the wrists and elbows, reach behind you (the shape of your chair permitting) and extend your arms as far back as they will comfortably go. Hold them in this position for 3 or 4 seconds, stretch, then return them to your lap. Keep your back as straight as possible during these movements. Repeat the entire cycle several times, moving briskly from one position to the next.

• Place your hands on your shoulders. Rapidly extend your arms upward, down, up, down. Do 25 touches in quick succession.

• Clasp your hands behind your head. Bend both elbows back as far as they will comfortably go, getting a good stretch in your shoulders and upper back. (You may wish to move a bit forward in your seat before you begin this exercise.) Hold for 20 seconds (or as long as the movement is comfortable), then return. Repeat several times.

• Extend your arms in front of you, palms upward. Make tight fists. Curl both arms in toward your chest, as if curling barbells, being sure to tighten and to place tension on the forearms and biceps. Repeat 25 times.

• Extend your arms in front of you. Open and close both hands rapidly 20 times.

• Extend your arms in front of you and make them into fists. Extend the fingers of each hand one at a time, first the thumb, then the index, middle, ring, and pinky, all in rapid sequence. Now reverse the sequence, closing the pinky first, then the ring finger, middle, index, and thumb. Repeat 5 times on each hand. With the right hand, bend your left hand back at the wrist as far as it will go, then reverse hands and repeat. Finally, shake both hands for 30 seconds.

• Place your hands on the side rails of the wheelchair and grip the pads. Push yourself upward as far as possible, as if doing a sitting pushup. Hold in this position for several beats, then slowly let yourself down again. Repeat this maneuver as many times as you can throughout the day. Pushing in this way will strengthen your arms and upper torso. It will relieve the weight on your buttocks, reducing the possibility of chafing and pressure sores.

• Grab your left shoulder with your right hand, your right shoulder with your left hand. Inch your fingers back on the shoulders as far as they will go. Remaining in this position, carefully rotate your torso first to the right and then the left 5 times to each side.

• Sit straight in the chair. With your upper back, neck, and head, extend the upper part of your spine toward the ceiling; at the same time, pull downward on the lower part of your spine. This two-way tension will produce a warm, stimulating stretch along your entire spine. Hold the tension for approximately 10 seconds, then release. Take a deep breath. Repeat several times, sensing the energy flow throughout the spine each time.

• Press and arch your lower back against the back of the chair. Hold for several beats, then reverse, arching your body forward and protruding your stomach. Make sure to get a firm stretch in both directions. Alternate back and forth slowly 10 times.

• Imagine that you are holding a paddle in both hands. Lean to one side of your "boat" and row. Do 10 strokes to one side, 10 to the other. Alternate sides until your shoulder and elbow joints feel pleasantly worked.

• Imagine that you are holding a rope in both hands. Pull the rope toward you to your left side for several beats, then to the right side. Continue to alternate sides.

• Imagine that you are holding the steering wheel of a car. Turn the wheel sharply to the right 10 times, then to the left 10 times. Continue to alternate directions, 10 times each way. Give a good stretch to your shoulder joints and elbows.

• Crook your arms. Pull them backward as if to touch your elbows together behind your back. This movement will cause your chest to protrude, providing a good stretch to the shoulders and upper back. Hold this position for 10 seconds, then reverse, moving your elbows forward until they are aligned one over the other in front of your chest, touching if possible. Hold here for another 10 seconds, then reverse (on the forward motion you may wish to alternate elbow positions, right over left one time, left over right the next). Alternate between backward and forward motions 10 times. Then release and relax.

• Sit up straight with your hands on your lap. Reach your right arm across your body, stretching it as far as it will comfortably go over your left knee. Hold for 5 seconds, then return to the starting position. Do 3 or 4 successive extensions, then reverse arms and perform the same movement to the opposite side. This exercise will give good extension on the intercostal muscles above the ribs and will help loosen up the trunk area.

• Lean forward. Clasp your hands behind your back. Raise them as high as they will go behind you, keeping your arms as straight as possible. Hold this position for at least 10 seconds, then release. Repeat several times.

• With the left arm extended straight out to the side, imagine that you are about to shoot a bow and arrow. Imagine that your left hand is gripping the bow while your right is slowly pulling back the string. As you pull, get plenty of tension and stretch on the right arm, and turn your head in sync with the movement, keeping your eyes on your right elbow as it pulls back to the right (at the end of the stretch you should be looking directly over your right shoulder). Now reverse directions, holding the bow in your right hand and pulling the string with your left hand (your head should now end up looking over your left shoulder). Alternate directions several times.

• Shrug your shoulders vigorously 20 times. Relax. Then push your shoulders rapidly forward, backward, forward, backward until they feel comfortably tired. You can repeat this movement anytime during the day. It will relax and loosen your whole upper torso.

• Rotate your right shoulder 10 times, making a kind of 360-degree circle at the joint. Then reverse directions. Repeat with the left shoulder. Do several alternations.

• Crane and stretch your neck as far up as it will comfortably go. Hold in this position for at least 10 seconds. Release and relax. Repeat this movement several times and do it throughout the day.

• Tilt your head as far to the right as it will comfortably go, trying to touch your right ear to your right shoulder. Repeat to the left. Get a good stretch in the lateral neck muscles, but be careful not to strain. Repeat 5 times to each side.

• Rotate your head clockwise and then counterclockwise several times. A relaxing variation on this movement is to let your neck go limp and rotate your head in a slow, easy motion, allowing it to drop of its own accord first to the front, then around to the right, then to the back, then to the left, and so on around in several successive rotations. Let gravity do most of the work for you. Do this exercise whenever you feel anxious and tense.

• *Resistive exercises*—If your doctor approves, you may wish to add a degree of difficulty to the above exercises by wearing cuff weights on your wrists or weighted boots on your feet. Both items can be purchased at any store that sells athletic equipment or sporting goods. If you wish you can make your own weighted cuffs, filling cloth bags with sand, sewing them up, and fastening them to your hands or feet.

Weight added to the limbs makes you work harder against the force of gravity, producing corresponding gains in strength, endurance, and muscle tone. Weight-lifting routines are also available for wheelchair patients. Speak to a physical therapist about developing a lifting routine specifically geared to your physical needs and endurance level.

Here are some exercise dos and don'ts for wheelchair-bound MS persons:

• DO practice the above exercises any time the spirit moves you. Five minutes here, 5 there add up to a lot at the end of the day and will keep you refreshed. The neck, shoulder, arm, and upper-torso exercises can all be done while watching TV, when talking to a friend, when sitting alone—whatever.

• DO ask your physical therapist what type of cushion is best to use while exercising. For some persons a soft pillow is best, for others a hard mat.

• DON'T exercise when you are tired or stressed.

• DO let vigorous exercise become a part of your daily or every-other-day routine.

• DO check to make sure that all the wheels on your chair are locked when you are exercising.

• DO drink plenty of water before and after every exercise session.

• DON'T eat for at least one hour before you begin exercising.

• DO empty your bladder before beginning each exercise session.

• DO ask for help when you need it. Don't be a hero.

Exercises for the Bedbound

A special note for caregivers: Patients suffering from the end stages of severe MS are often confined to bed. Now more than ever, exercise is essential, not only for the usual health reasons—circulation, metabolism, etc.—but to prevent cramping, curvature of the spine, atrophy of muscle tone, contractures (shortening of the ligaments and tendons), and pressure sores.

Bedbound patients are often severely movement-restricted and will usually have to be helped through the exercises. The following movements can all be done with a caregiver's assistance:

• With the patient on his or her back, lift the right arm and pull it gently toward you, giving a good stretch to the arm and shoulder joint. Repeat with the left arm. Alternate several times on each side.

• With the patient on his or her back, lift the right arm straight up and rotate it in its socket several times, both directions, moving it through its full range of motion. Repeat with the left. Alternate several times.

• With the patient on his or her back, lift the right arm back and over the head (keeping it parallel to the floor). Gently pull, stretch, and rotate the arm in each direction, being careful not to apply undue pressure to the shoulder joint. Release. Repeat with the left arm. Alternate several times between arms.

• With the patient on his or her back, lift the right arm straight up and rotate the hand, both directions, through the full 360-degree range of motion. Repeat with the left arm. Alternate several times.

• Have the patient wiggle the fingers vigorously. Have the patient perform this motion without assistance throughout the day.

• With the patient on his or her back, lift the right leg, pull it toward you gently but firmly for several moments, then release. Repeat with the left leg. Alternate between legs several times.

• With the patient on his or her back, lift the right leg and rotate the foot, both directions, through its full range of motion. Repeat with the left leg. Alternate between legs several times.

• With the patient on his or her back, lift the right leg and rotate it as fully as possible at the hip joint, both directions, through the complete range of motion. Repeat with the left leg. Alternate between legs several times.

• With the patient on his or her back, bend the right leg at the knee, press it down to the chest, hold in this position for several moments, then release. Repeat with the left leg. Do several alternations.

• With the patient on his or her back, ask the patient to lift his or her legs several inches up from the bed (if possible) and wiggle the toes vigorously. Instruct the patient to perform this exercise as frequently during the day as possible.

• With the patient on his or her back, lift the right leg and move it diagonally across to the left side, stretching it as far as it will comfortably go. Maintain this extension for several moments, then release. Repeat with the left leg. Do several repetitions on both legs, being careful not to press or pull with too much force.

• With the patient on his or her back and the caregiver standing at the head of the bed, lift the patient's head off the pillow and gently pull it toward you, lifting the shoulders as well (if feasible). Hold in this position for several moments, giving a good hyperextension to the neck and cervical areas of the spine. Then release. Repeat several times.

• Ask the patient to tighten his or her abdominal muscles for 5 to 10 seconds several times in a row. You can massage this part of the patient's body, kneading the flesh and making gentle circular motions in the center of the abdomen.

• Direct the patient to move his or her hips from side to side. Repeat several times.

• Ask the patient to take 5 or 6 deep, full breaths. Encourage the patient to practice slow, deep breathing throughout the day.

Caregivers should take note of these important concerns for exercising bedbound patients:

• When handling patients' limbs, grip them firmly but gently, not too tight, not too loose. Ask the patient if your grip is comfortable before beginning any movement.

• If a particular joint is painful, do not grip it directly. Cradle the area immediately above it and below it. For example, if there is pain in a patient's knee, grip the upper calf and lower thigh while moving the leg.

• Before you begin moving a patient's limb, explain to the patient what you are about to do, and why. For example [taking the patient's hand]: "Okay, Ralph. Now I'm going to pull your arm straight up and over your head. This will give you a nice stretch on your arms and shoulders. Try to relax while I'm doing it" [performs the maneuver]. "Now I'm going to stretch the other arm. Okay? This will feel good in your shoulder."

• If spasticity occurs while you are exercising a person's limbs, stop the movement for a moment and apply gentle pressure directly to the spastic part. The muscle will soon relax. Then continue.

• Never rush an exercise session. Move bedbound patients through their routine with steady, gentle, rhythmic motions. Avoid all sudden jerks, pulls, or surprises. When movements are rapid or abrupt they can induce spasticity.

• Never force a joint beyond its comfortable range of motion. Easy does it—always.

• Incorporate exercise into the bedbound person's regular activities of daily living. Encourage patients (if possible) to roll in the bed from side to side several times a day, to button their own cuffs, brush their teeth, comb their hair, wash their faces, feed themselves. All of these movements constitute exercise of a sort.

When putting on shirts, encourage patients to stretch their arms over their heads and hold this position for several moments. When putting on shoes and socks, have them bend down and touch their toes in the process. When watching TV, encourage patients to rotate their hands and wiggle their toes. When reading a book, patients can hunch their shoulders and rotate their necks. Encourage frequent stretching while in bed.

• Always know a bedbound patient's physical limits and never exceed them. If you have any questions along these lines, consult with the patient's physician before beginning any exercise program.

MASSAGE FOR THE BEDBOUND

A really helpful auxiliary measure caregivers can add to the regular exercise routine is a daily or every-other-day session of body massage.

Massage helps circulation, stimulates the lymph glands, improves skin tone, and aids elimination. It also offers moments of intimate contact between caregiver and patient, an encounter that can do a lot toward raising a bedbound person's spirits and making him or her feel loved and important.

Gentle, firm, and slow are the orders of the day here. Use a good massage oil or skin cream. Start at the feet and work up to the head. The standard strokes used for massage include:

• *Kneading*—The most basic of massage techniques, kneading involves the deep manipulation of muscle tissue by means of folding and pressing with the fingers and thumbs, not unlike the way one kneads bread.

• *Effleurage*—Long, continuous stroking movements delivered along the entire length of the person's limbs, back, and torso. This technique is done with both hands simultaneously, often with one palm placed on top of the other. Its benefits include increased lymphatic drainage, relaxation of muscle tissue, and improved circulation.

• *Friction*—Brisk buffing and rubbing movements on the skin surface, often delivered without benefit of oil to increase friction. Friction rub helps open the pores, bring blood to the skin, and produce tone and color to the skin.

• *Percussion*—Tapping, light slapping, drumming on the body surface. Percussion breaks up muscular congestion, relieves muscle spasms, relaxes strain.

• *Vibration*—The fingers are placed over the body surface and vibrated. This technique takes a little practice. Once mastered it helps stimulate blood flow and nerve force.

7

Health Maintenance Guide for Persons with MS

People with MS think differently about their health than those who do not have the disease. Disease-free persons can often afford to push the envelope a bit now and then, to drink a little too much, to keep late hours, to become overweight, to avoid exercise. Time is on their side while they are young. Later on the piper will have to be paid, no doubt, but for the time being a healthy young person's body will remain more or less intact, if not strong and fit, despite the insults inflicted on it.

This is not the case for MS persons. "I notice that every time I get a little cold or sniffles," one patient says, "my symptoms start acting up. I've been told that when MS people get sick they get *more* sick than others. I believe it. And God help me if I really get sick or don't take care of myself. I've had three or four flareups that have come while I was badly laid up, making me miserable and throwing me back a lot of pegs. It took me an age to build myself back up. Now I'm very careful."

Forewarned is forearmed. In this chapter we will review some of the critical steps MS persons can take, not only to avoid becoming sick but to strengthen their bodies and to steel themselves against the infections and health hazards to which they are especially vulnerable.

You may already know some of the information presented in this chapter. If this is the case, that's good. It means you are an alert and well-informed patient. Just make sure to put your knowledge into practice whenever you can.

Others, however, may not be as well versed in the principles of general health maintenance, and this chapter is especially for them.

If you fall into this second category, know that by following a majority of the recommendations offered here you will see results both in your sense of physical well-being and, just as important, in your mental and emotional life. A wholesome regime of sensible living invariably helps both the body and mind of MS persons, giving them the confidence and optimism so necessary for dealing with their disease.

THE IMPORTANCE OF DIET

Enough has been written about diet and MS to fill this book and several others. William A. Sibley's classic work on MS, *Therapeutic Claims in Multiple Sclerosis* (New York, Demos Publications, 1988) devotes dozens of pages to summarizing the dietary "cures" for MS that have been put forward through the years. Some of these approaches have been propounded by legitimate clinical researchers, men and women of sincere intent who have spent many years delving into the relationship between what we eat and how it affects neurological functioning. Other theories fall into the category of nonorthodox medicine, though they too are often put forward by intelligent, careful researchers. Still others deserve only the title of quackery.

Over the past decades, for example, the following dietary

regimes have been suggested as being either beneficial for MS patients or directly curative:

• *Aloe vera treatment*—Extracting the juice from the aloe vera plant, a common succulent, and taking it orally several times a day for its dietary benefits.

• *Cerebrosides treatment*—Taking the fatty acids from beef cerebrosides—cerebrosides are fatty lipids found in the brain and central nervous system—and using them as a dietary supplement.

• *The Cambridge liquid diet*—A low-calorie diet often used for treating obesity.

• *Sucrose and tobacco elimination diet*—A dietary regimen that eliminates all sugars and tobacco, based on the notion that multiple sclerosis is caused by an allergy to these substances.

• *Gluten-free diet*—Gluten is a form of protein found in wheat and rye. Since MS occurs mostly in countries that thrive on food products made from these grains, it is reasoned that their elimination from the diet will eliminate MS.

• *Raw-food diet*—A dietary regime designed to build up the body's natural immunities to the MS virus. It is comprised of uncooked, unprocessed, fresh-picked fruits and vegetables (minus some forms of lettuce), plus unprocessed dairy products, selected meats, and whole grains.

The above is just a sampling. There are many others. How much do these and other dietary regimes help?

According to the International Federation of Multiple Sclerosis Societies and the National Multiple Sclerosis Society, not at all. Both these organizations concur in their judgment that no dietary regime *of any kind* has provided substantial clinical evidence of controlling the symptoms of MS or of curing the disease. The many documented cases of people who have followed such diets and had symptom relief (or even experienced complete disease elimination) are, according to these organizations, anecdotal.

More than likely a remission of symptoms would have occurred naturally for these patients no matter what foods they ate or potions they drank.

Does this mean then that diet plays no part in MS?

Perhaps. But perhaps not.

Certainly it seems counterproductive to follow the more extreme dietary regimens; and in many cases people who put their undying faith in such theories are fortifying themselves with false hopes. At the same time, a sound and nourishing diet is essential to the physical upkeep of MS patients and should be a high priority on everyone's list. Moreover, although the testimonials reported by patients who have profited from dietary approaches remain on the hearsay level, many doctors and medical professionals have noted definite improvements in patients who employed a careful dietary approach, and a number of them have now concluded that diet does play some part, at least, in the MS story.

Finally, there is the placebo effect to consider: If persons believe strongly enough in dietary cures they may, through some physiomental process not entirely understood, experience beneficial results. Whether or not these benefits are a natural part of the relapsing-remitting disease process or whether they are caused by the powers of belief is irrelevant. If it works, keep doing it.

So where does this leave us?

Simply with the understanding that a sound, wholesome diet is a prerequisite for all MS persons no matter what their degree of debilitation. And further that if MS persons decide they want to try a particular dietary regime—and assuming that this regime does not produce malnutrition, extreme weight loss, or other dangerous side effects—there is no reason why they should not do so. The following points of information will all be helpful.

REAL NUTRITION: WHAT IS IT?

Three square meals a day. But what does it mean?

Essentially, that all of us should eat meals that are properly balanced between the three main food groups: carbohydrates, fats, and proteins.

While it's true that terms like "fats," "carbohydrate diet," "protein supplements," and others have become familiar parts of our language, most people have incomplete notions of why these substances are nourishing, and even what they are in the first place.

Quite simply, carbohydrates, fats, and proteins are the basic organic chemical compounds that we call "nutrients." Along with vitamins, minerals, and water, they comprise the full range of food-stuffs that nourish and sustain the human body. Just about every liquid and solid we consume contains one or more of these, and almost every function that our bodies perform is dependent on a steady input of them for good health.

Known as the "large nutrients" (as opposed to vitamins and minerals, which are called the "small nutrients"), carbohydrates, fats, and proteins are broken down in the stomach and intestines, absorbed through the intestinal wall, and passed into the bloodstream. Eventually they are transported by the blood to trillions of hungry cells throughout the body, where they are put to work to form new tissue, stored for future use, metabolized for energy, and used to provide fuel for any number of regulatory body processes. A combination of all three large nutrients is vitally necessary for the maintenance of health.

Here's a brief rundown of which foods fall into which nutrient category:

Fats

Fats are mainly components of dairy products, meat, nuts, eggs, and certain legumes such as peanuts. Oil is exclusively a fatty substance.

A breakdown of the percent of fat in fat-containing foods looks like this:

FAT AND CHOLESTEROL CONTENT IN COMMON FOODS

Food (100-gram serving)	Total Fat Content (in Grams)	Cholesterol (in Milligrams)
Beef (cooked)	6.1	91
Lamb (cooked)	7	100
Chicken (light meat, cooked, without skin)	4	85
Chicken (dark meat, cooked, without skin)	9.7	93
Turkey	3.2	69
Pork (cooked)	30	89
Hot dog (all-beef)	30	51
Salmon, pink (canned)	6	35
Tuna in oil (canned)	8	65
Tuna in water (canned)	.8	63
Lobster	1.5	85
Eggs	12	551
Cream, Half and Half	11	37
Cream, heavy	35	110
Milk, 1%	1.2	4
Milk, whole	4	14
Cheese, American	31	94
Cheese, cheddar	33	105
Cheese, cottage (creamed)	4	15
Cheese, cottage (dry-curd)	.4	7
Cheese, parmesan	30	79
Cheese, Swiss	27	92
Butter	81	220
Margarine	80	0

FAT AND CHOLESTEROL CONTENT IN COMMON FOODS *(Continued)*

Food (100-gram serving)	Total Fat Content (in Grams)	Cholesterol (in Milligrams)
Mayonnaise	80	0
Yogurt, plain (low-fat)	5	6
Ice cream, vanilla	11	45
Ice milk	4	14
Sherbet	2	7
Walnuts	64	0
Cashews	46	0
Olives	13	0
Oil, corn	100	0
Oil, cottonseed	100	0
Oil, olive	100	0
Oil, safflower	100	0
Oil, sesame	100	0
Lard	100	95

In this century consumption of dietary fat has risen at rather amazing rates, so that today it accounts on the average for 40 percent of our daily nutritive intake. With new scientific evidence showing that high-fat diets lead to harmful cholesterol formation and overweight, things are changing, and fat intake is decreasing in this country every year. Some medical researchers, moreover, believe that an as yet unknown relationship exists between reduced fat content in the diet and improvement of MS symptoms, although this theory has yet to be clinically established.

It is presently recommended by the American Heart Association that dietary fats constitute no more than 30 percent (and far better, 10 or 15 percent) of our daily diet.

Carbohydrates

Despite increased consumption of fats and proteins in the West, carbohydrates still make up the majority of most people's diets

---

In a nutshell, a standard low-fat diet includes:

- No more than three servings a week of a low-fat meat such as chicken or turkey. Deep-sea fish such as flounder, sole, or scrod can be eaten any time.
- Plenty of fresh vegetables for lunch and dinner.
- Use low-fat dairy products: skim or 1 percent milk, low-fat yogurt, buttermilk, curd cottage cheese, skimmed mozzarella and ricotta cheese.
- Use polyunsaturated oils in salads and for cooking. These include corn oil, safflower oil, sesame oil, soybean oil, and sunflower oil.
- Eat no more than one or two eggs a week.
- Eat plenty of whole-wheat grains. Shop for dietary-style breads.
- Avoid sweets, beef, pork, lamb, high-fat dairy foods, fried foods, and the high-fat foods in general listed above.

---

and are the body's main supply of fuel. Typical eaters at the American and European table take in 200 pounds of carbohydrates for every 20 pounds of protein. And this is as it should be, for tissue building and energy production are both dependent on these substances, as is the proper functioning of the nerve cells. Appearing in two forms, the easily digestible simple carbohydrates (such as grapes, corn, greens) and the more slowly digested starches or complex carbohydrates (such as grains and legumes), carbohydrates are also the major conveyor of fiber into the diet, a boon to both digestion and fat elimination. Indeed, without an adequate supply of these energy foods into the body, the brain malfunctions and the nervous system shuts down.

Simple carbohydrates are found in sweet fruits such as pears, apples, guavas, berries, pineapples, and plums, and in vegetables such as tomatoes, lettuce, squash, beets, turnips, and cucumbers. Complex carbohydrates appear in grains: wheat, corn, oats, rye, barley, millet, and rice. They are also found in bananas, potatoes, legumes, and, to a limited extent, in dairy products.

In general, it is recommended that at least 55 percent of a

person's diet, and hopefully as much as 80 percent, be made up of complex carbohydrates.

Protein

Dietary protein is found in meat, dairy products, legumes, and to a limited extent in grains (wheat grain, for instance, measures approximately 20 percent protein). Containing the eight varieties of essential amino acids not produced within the body, protein is the very stuff of cell building and regeneration, responsible for the manufacture of new tissue and the repair of old, for neutralizing and distributing body water, and for maintaining the pH balance in bodily fluids between acidic and alkaline. Many enzymes are produced from the end products of food proteins, and hemoglobin itself is protein-based. Muscle, hair, the kidneys and liver, the tendons, the nerves—all are forged from this essential material.

At the same time, it is now believed that dietary protein has been oversold to the American public, and that too much of it is as bad as not enough. Excess protein intake can produce an overabundance of nitrogenous and sulfurous wastes. Both the kidneys and the liver become enlarged as a result, and in extreme cases disabled. Excess animal protein has a tendency to produce acids that steal vital calcium salts from the blood. This leads to a weakening of the skeletal structure and ultimately to spontaneous bone fractures. So be sparing. Meat and cheese three times a day is definitely discouraged.

It is likewise a fallacy to assume that protein produces "instant energy," as we are sometimes told. The public once heard a good deal about athletes eating enormous steaks before a game or of competitors stuffing themselves on protein supplements. In fact, protein tends to produce energy over the long run, not the short; carbohydrates, and specifically the natural sugars found in fruit and vegetables, bring energy to the system a good deal faster and more effectively than protein. In terms of multiple sclerosis sufferers, this means that during periods of fatigue a sweet apple or pear, a bowl of fresh vegetables, or a glass of fruit juice is more likely to generate revival than a protein-based food or supplement.

In general, it is recommended that a person's diet include no more than 10 to 15 percent protein a day.

To review, the overall recommended balance between the three basic food families is:

- 15 to 20 percent fats
- 70 to 75 percent carbohydrates
- 10 percent protein

Here are some eating tips specifically tailored for persons with MS:

• *Eat plenty of fiber*—Constipation is a common problem among MS persons and will be discussed later in this chapter. For the time being, know that one of the principal ways in which this problem can be avoided, or at least reduced, is by cutting down on constipation-producing foods—fatty meats, chocolate, fried foods, sweets, and alcohol—and by increasing the amount of fiber taken into the diet.

One of the insidious side effects of constipation is that when fecal residues remain in the system for long periods of time they tend to stagnate in the colon. Certain kinds of bacteria, bifidobacteria in particular, are then given the chance to breed. Bifidobacteria contain enzymes that transmute bile salts into toxic residue if allowed to remain in the intestines too long, and their prolonged residence in the digestive tract should be avoided.

Fiber's ability to prevent constipation is well known, and with good reason. Fiber exerts a strong absorbent action in the intestines, drawing local stores of water into the feces and swelling their size and weight. These stores add both bulk and softness to the stool, and help it transit more swiftly through the digestive tract. Tests show that persons who favor a high-fiber diet eliminate more frequently than those who do not; that their feces are larger and fuller; and that more wastes are excreted at every elimination. Foods with high fiber content should therefore be a fundamental part of the diet of every MS person. A list of high-fiber foods is worth posting in your kitchen:

FIBER CONTENT IN COMMON FOODS

Food	Amount	Dietary Fiber Grams per Serving
Apple	1 whole	3.0
Asparagus	4 spears	.9
Avocado	1 whole	4.4
Banana	1 whole	1.8
Beets	1 cup	4.2
Bran	1 cup	23.0
Broccoli	1 cup	2.2
Cabbage	1 cup	2.2
Cantaloupe	½ fruit	1.6
Carrots	1 cup	2.1
Cauliflower	1 cup	2.2
Corn	1 ear on cob	5.9
Cracked-wheat bread	1 slice	2.1
Cucumber	1 ounce	0.1
Figs	1 medium-sized	2.4
Grapefruit	½ cup	0.6
Grapes	12	0.3
Green beans	1 cup	3.9
Green pepper	1	0.8
Grits	½ cup	0.1
Kidney beans	1 cup	2.0
Lentil soup	1 cup	5.5
Lettuce	1 serving	1.5
Mango	1 fruit	3.0
Mushrooms	1 cup	1.8
Okra	½ cup	2.6
Orange	1 fruit	2.5
Parsnips	1 cup	6.2
Peach	1 fruit	1.4
Pear	1 fruit	2.6
Peas	1 cup	7.9
Pickle, dill	1 whole	1.2
Pineapple	1 cup	2.2

FIBER CONTENT IN COMMON FOODS *(Continued)*

Food	Amount	Dietary Fiber Grams per Serving
Plums	1 fruit	0.2
Potato, baked in the skin	1 whole	3.0
Prunes	1	1.0
Pumpernickel bread	1 slice	1.2
Radish	5	0.2
Raisins	2 tablespoons	1.2
Raspberries	1 cup	9.2
Rice, brown	1 cup	1.1
Rice, white	1 cup	0.4
Rolled oats	½ cup	4.5
Spinach	1 cup	11.4
Strawberries	1 cup	3.4
Tomato	1 whole	2.1
Watercress	1 serving	0.7
Whole-wheat bread	1 slice	2.4

Patients can supplement their fiber intake each day by eating a serving of wheat- or oat-bran fiber. There is some evidence, not fully corroborated, that oat bran reduces the amount of cholesterol in the system and lowers overall blood fats, so it may serve several purposes at once.

Bran can be purchased in bulk or found in foods such as bran cereals and muffins. Add it to sauces, cereals, and gravies as a thickener, or sprinkle whole-bran supplements on top of cereal and yogurt desserts.

• *Avoid overly processed foods*—One painless way to naturally increase the intake of fiber is by eating foods that are not heavily processed and refined.

Bread is a good place to begin. Modern milling machines used by commercial bakers not only remove the outer layers of the individual grain but the delicate inner skin too, the aleurone layer, which is the most digestible and nutritious part of the food. Studies have shown that at least 50 percent of nutrients are removed by processing wheat and a healthy portion of the bulk and fiber as well. Bread from unrefined flour is available in supermarkets as well as in bakeries and health-food stores; in terms of nutritional assets and benefits to the digestion it is worth the extra money.

As with wheat, the less rice is refined the more nutrients and fiber remain. The part of the grain removed in polishing, the bran coat, contains 10 percent of rice's protein, 75 percent of its minerals, and most of its roughage. Brown rice is available today in supermarkets and health-food stores.

In general, go with foods that are fresh, wholesome, and unprocessed.

• *Avoid animal fat*—Although nothing has been proven to date, many physicians and researchers have noted that MS patients tend to do better when their intake of animal fats is kept at a minimum; this includes meat and dairy products in particular.

It has, for instance, been pointed out that in societies where the diet is low in animal fats, populations show a lower incidence of MS than in countries where dietary fats are abundant. Reporting on studies of MS patients who have followed a restricted-fat diet for an average of seventeen years, Dr. William Sibley *(Therapeutic Claims in Multiple Sclerosis)* reports that a slower rate of progression, fewer exacerbations, and lower death rates were all reported, compared to the normal course of MS as described in neurological literature. Sibley adds that no matched control group was looked at concurrently in the study, and that as yet many physicians are dubious concerning its basic hypothesis. He concludes that although the low-fat diet has not been proven to be effective in the treatment of MS it is relatively free of adverse side effects during long-term use, and "the possibility of a partial or incomplete effect has not been excluded."

Taking all things into consideration, therefore—the many anecdotal tales of patients who have improved by avoiding fats, the demographic indications, clinical studies that suggest the diet's effectiveness, and the not inconsiderable fact that a diet low in animal fat is generally good for persons no matter what their state of health—it can be said that there is no reason not to follow a low-fat diet and several important ones in its favor.

• *Increase your liquid intake*—Increased amounts of liquids taken daily will help control constipation, keep the body hydrated, flush out wastes, and generally improve the working of the entire physical system.

Take plenty of fruit juices during the day. Mix them with seltzer or bubbling water for added taste. Coffee and tea are okay, though in moderation (while most MS patients report no adverse effects from coffee drinking, a few do; experiment). Eight to ten glasses of liquid a day should be the goal.

Note, however, that in certain cases increased liquid intake can pose a dilemma. If an MS person suffers bladder complications and already has problems of retention and frequency, liquids may need to be limited rather than increased, especially at night for those prone to nocturia. Multiple sclerosis patients who suffer from bladder disorders should consult with their physicians for advice on this issue.

While on the subject of bladder difficulties and liquid intake, it should also be mentioned that many doctors and nutritionists recommend a daily intake of cranberry juice for persons who suffer frequent urinary infections. Cranberry juice is a powerful specific for acidifying the body's supply of urine. Acid urine discourages the growth of harmful bacteria and is potentially an easy and tasty form of prevention against infection. Again, consult with your physician if you have any questions or hesitations along these lines.

• *Vitamins*—As with diets, there have been many theories set forth concerning the relationship between MS and vitamins, most of them linking MS to some sort of vitamin deficiency. Such theories were propounded as far back as the 1920s and they continue to pop up today. In fact, at various times in the past more than *half* of all the thirteen basic vitamins—A, C, D, E, K, and B_{12} plus the B-complex vitamins to be exact—have been championed as possible aids for this disease.

But be careful. Proponents of vitamin cures often place their patients on potentially dangerous doses of megavitamins, sometimes for extended periods of time. One megavitamin regime, for instance, recommends that subjects ingest massive amounts of each of the major vitamins to make up for their reputed deficiency, even though it is understood by every informed medical professional that overmedication of a vitamin such as A can cause a condition known as *hypervitaminosis A,* which not only weakens the already fatigued MS patient but causes symptoms such as nausea, loss of appetite, dry skin, hair loss, irregular menstruation, and in extreme cases enlargement of the liver. Too much vitamin D will also produce problems, specifically weakness, depression, and increased urination, three symptoms that plague many MS sufferers already.

The fact of the matter is, no one has yet produced clinical evidence of any kind showing either that MS is caused by a vitamin deficiency or that taking massive doses of vitamins improves a patient's overall condition.

At the same time, vitamins are essential nutrients for the healthy working of the human organism, and with few exceptions (such as vitamin D), the body cannot produce them internally and must ingest them through food substances. It is thus important that MS patients eat a diet that includes a proper share of these basic chemicals. A nutshell review of vitamins and the foods they are found in follows below. Note before studying it that there are two types of vitamins: the fat-soluble family, A, D, E, and K, which are taken in with fats and stored for periods of time in the liver; and the water-soluble vitamins, C and the B-complex vitamins, which remain in the body for brief periods of time and are then excreted.

What about taking vitamin supplements? A good multiple vitamin may be of value and can be taken with reasonable doses of minerals as well. Anecdotally, some MS patients report feeling better from these substances. Again, it can't hurt to try, but only as long as the doses are within the recommended limits.

VITAMIN CONTENT OF FOODS

Vitamin	*Sources*
Oil-soluble	
Vitamin A	Eggs, fish, liver, and certain vegetables, such as carrots
Vitamin D	Dairy products, fish, liver, eggs, vegetable oil, eggs
Vitamin E	Meat, wheat germ, green leafy vegetables, vegetable oils, nuts, eggs
Vitamin K	Turnips, broccoli, vegetable oils, dairy products, meat
Water-soluble	
Vitamin C	Leafy vegetables, citrus fruits, berries, melons, papayas
Biotin	Organ meats, eggs, citrus fruits, melons, dried beans
Folic acid	Green leafy vegetables, organ meats, eggs, grains, nuts, peas
Niacin	Meat, chicken, turkey, fish, grains, dried beans, peas
Pantothenic acid	Organ meats, eggs, brewer's yeast, vegetables, grains
Pyridoxine	Meats, dried beans, peanuts, bananas, grains
Riboflavin	Meat, dairy products, eggs, grains, leafy vegetables
Thiamine	Grains, beans, nuts, fish, meat, whole-wheat bread
Vitamin B_{12}	Meat and dairy products

• *Dietary food supplements*—The wide array of food and mineral supplements recommended at one time or another for MS such as choline, lecithin, aloe vera, primrose oil, thyroid extract, calcium lactate, brewer's yeast, Chinese herb preparations, etc., may or may not improve a well person's general state of health, but they seem to make no difference in MS—with one *possible* exception: fish oil.

Fish-oil therapy began years ago when researchers observed that Eskimo tribes in northern Canada and Alaska consume enormous amounts of blubber and fish oil every year, yet show a considerably lower incidence of many of the diseases that plague people in the temperate climates, especially heart disease and atherosclerosis. On the list of low-incidence diseases also was multiple sclerosis.

Researchers discovered that certain fish oils have an inhibiting effect on tissue inflammation, and from this they reasoned that the inflammation produced by demyelination may respond positively to fish-oil supplements. Several studies were launched in Great Britain to determine the therapeutic effectiveness of this substance. Though the findings did not reach the level of statistical significance for MS, they were substantial enough to cause the Therapeutic Claims Committee of the International Federation of Multiple Sclerosis Societies to go on record as saying that fish-oil therapy may have *some* efficacy in improving the disease.

Since, in fact, fish oils have no negative side effects of any significance except perhaps their unpleasant smell, it may be worth experimenting with them. Fish oils are sold at most pharmacies and health-food stores, and are relatively inexpensive. Try them for several months and see if any improvement is forthcoming.

Another oil that may have some value in this regard, it should be mentioned, is sunflower seed oil, an unsaturated fatty acid. Several lab tests plus a great deal of anecdotal evidence have shown through the years that linoleic acid, a substance that abounds in sunflower seed oil, is useful in strengthening the immune system and normalizing its functions. Best used in uncooked form, sunflower seed oil can be added to salads, mixed with juice, or taken directly by the spoonful. Like fish oil, it represents a painless dietary option that contains no hidden liabilities and several *possible* assets.

DEALING WITH CONSTIPATION

Constipation—infrequent or difficult bowel movements—is generally more a symptom than a disease. Depending on circumstances, it can be triggered by stress, depression, poor eating habits, insufficient exercise, reaction to medications, inadequate fluid intake—or the MS itself. Though occasionally caused by demyelination of the nerve fibers controlling the organs of elimination, however, constipation is more commonly a result of the psychological reactions and the sedentary living habits that MS tends to encourage.

In many instances, moreover, though the number of bowel movements that a person makes is reduced, MS fecal incontinence is rare, and at worst patients find themselves eliminating every several days or even once a week rather than once or twice daily. Though unpleasant, this is not cause for alarm and is usually a lifestyle modification that people can live with.

In cases of chronic constipation, the first line of defense is a natural one: proper diet, plenty of dietary fiber, and supplementary doses of bran.

Start with proper diet. This means both addition and subtraction: addition of high-fiber foods, subtraction of low-fiber foods. We have already reviewed the subject of fiber earlier in the chapter, and readers should check with the chart listed there for information on fiber-bearing nutrients.

In general, patients will also want to eliminate from their meals any constipation-causing food such as chocolate, sweets, fatty meats, fried foods, and for some persons hot and spicy foods. Eat more fresh vegetables, fresh fruits, and foods that ferment quickly in the gut such as sauerkraut, sauerkraut juice, cabbage juice, sourdough bread, and pickles. For some people the addition of sauerkraut alone restores regularity. Sample a drink made up of half sauerkraut juice, half tomato juice, with a squeeze of lemon. If it helps, use it every day. Another good remedy is honey and lemon juice.

Meanwhile, avoid iced drinks and favor hot ones. Add to the diet natural laxative foods, such as yogurt, garlic, rhubarb, kefir, papaya juice, pumpkin seeds, prunes, prune juice, and ground flaxseed. Most can be purchased at a supermarket and the rest at any natural-food store, along with acidophilus milk, which in some persons increases abdominal fermentation in a dramatic way. Finally, try boiling a half-cup of wheat berries every day in water or milk until they are soft, then eat them with fruit or raisins first thing in the morning. Stay on this regime for at least a month—the effects may take a while to begin.

Other natural aids to prevent constipation include increased liquid intake, daily exercise, and self-massage of the abdomen. (Place your palms over your navel, one hand on top of the other. Press firmly. Move the hands in a clockwise motion, the direction in which the food passes through the digestive tract, applying deep, rhythmic pressure. Do this exercise several minutes in the morning and at night.) Dr. John K. Wolf in his worthy book *Mastering Multiple Sclerosis: A Guide to Management* (Academy Books: Rutland, Vermont, 1987) states that some MS patients find they can induce a bowel movement simply by scratching the skin located just above their anus. This area, Dr. Wolf explains, is connected to the sacral spinal cord segments that run to the rectum and anus, and for some people stimulating it produces nerve signals that encourage elimination.

If diet and other natural measures do not produce the desired effect, the next step is to try bran.

Bran is the chaff of the wheat or oat kernel removed during the refining process. Besides being a specific for constipation, it contains small amounts of vitamin B and trace minerals, and is both safe and tasty. If sprinkled over cereal, into a stew, or taken by the teaspoonful with a glass of water, it produces regularity in many MS people, even those who have suffered from constipation for years.

Bran works by absorbing water and expanding the size of

the feces, thus irritating the lining of the colon and increasing peristalsis. When used in moderation—several teaspoonfuls a day—it can be a powerful ally for regaining regularity. Do be careful of overuse, however, as excess amounts of bran in the digestive system may compact into large watery lumps, eventually obstructing the intestines and *producing* constipation rather than relieving it.

Finally, as a last resort, try laxatives.

Many members of the medical community look on over-the-counter laxatives as a necessary evil at best and a possible source of addiction at worst. Laxatives easily become habit-forming, and some varieties irritate the colon lining. They sap the vigor of the digestive system, and overuse can atrophy key digestive organs, causing the eliminative system to lose its ability to work properly without the stimulation of chemicals. Users may then find themselves caught up in a habit that is difficult to break.

Nevertheless, the use of laxatives is sometimes a necessity among MS users, and when it is begin with the most gentle variety, the so-called *bulk-forming laxatives*. Besides bran, these include psyllium derivatives such as Metamucil, Siblin, and Muci-lose; malt soup extracts like Maltsupex; and polycarbophil, which comes in Mitrolan tablets. Take these preparations with plenty of water, and expect to see results in a day or so.

If the bulk-forming laxatives don't do the trick, the next step up in effectiveness is the *stool softeners* such as Bu-Lax, D-S-S, and Colace. Take them only for a day or two at most. Glycerine suppositories can be helpful for some persons, as can the *lubricant laxatives*, such as mineral oil, though overdose of this substance will interfere with proper nutrient absorption (taking mineral oil at bedtime can occasionally cause older people to aspirate the oil from the stomach into the lungs). *Saline laxatives* such as milk of magnesia and tartar salts are another powerful bowel stimulator, though these can cause loss of important body salts and are not generally recommended.

The most powerful of all laxatives are the *stimulant laxatives*. These work directly on the intestines, artificially reducing the transit time food takes to work its way down through the bowels and out of the body. In this category you will find castor oil, bile salts, bisacodyl (Cenalax, Fleet Bisacodyl, Dulcolax), phenolph-thalein (Ex-Lax, Feen-A-Mint, Phenolax), cascara sagrada, and senna.

It is suggested that MS patients use stimulant laxatives only on the rarest occasions, and then only if impaction threatens or if absolutely none of the other alternatives mentioned above do the job. Never use them for more than three or four days at a time. They work too well—the bowels will quickly become dependent on them. If you have any questions about laxative use and consti-pation problems in general, consult with your physician.

DEALING WITH SLEEP PROBLEMS

Sleep disorders are not usually produced by the pathological changes caused by multiple sclerosis, yet a number of MS patients complain of insomnia or broken sleep patterns. Such problems, it appears on close examination, result not from the disease itself but from secondary factors such as tension, inactivity, and depression.

Read the testimony of several patients on the subject:

Iris P.: It's funny, because during the day I'm tired a lot and sometimes find myself nodding out; or while I'm at work I wish I could be home in bed, asleep. At night when I crawl under the covers I have the hardest time getting to sleep, and sometimes I'll lie there staring at the ceiling for hours and hours, even though my body feels bone-tired. There doesn't seem to be any connection the way there used to be between my tiredness and my ability to fall asleep.

Arnold D.: When I was a teenager my mother used to have to blow me out of bed mornings with a huge bomb. Since I've gotten multiple sclerosis it's become the opposite. I only sleep several hours a night now, and that's on the light side; practically any sound or light in the room and I'm wide awake, and then have trouble the rest of the evening getting back to sleep. My wife and I have had to move to separate rooms because my sleep is so "iffy" and up and down. Also, since my hip hurts—from the disease, I guess—each time I roll over there's a twitching pain there, and it keeps me up. If I don't roll on that side I start to feel uncomfortable, but if I do it keeps me up. I've used sleeping pills sometimes, but I don't want to become reliant on them. I just sweat it out.

Those who suffer sleep disturbances will be happy to learn that while insomnia is debilitating, it causes little or no permanent physical damage, even over extended periods of time. Most of us can go as long as seventy-two hours without closing our eyes and then make up the loss during several long sessions of undisturbed sleep. Test subjects have been kept awake for as long as two hundred hours without demonstrating permanent psychological change. The symptoms that do occur from insomnia—memory loss, vagueness, restlessness, depression, impairment of mental ability—are akin to symptoms that some MS persons experience, but they are deeper, more profound, and have a certain intense quality that we all recognize when we are deprived of sleep.

What may seem like a night of no sleep at all, moreover, is often a night of *light* sleep punctuated by continual dreaming. In an experiment carried out some time ago at a university sleep laboratory, a number of insomniacs were placed in special sleep rooms and asked to press a button whenever they heard a prearranged buzzing sound. Results showed that more often than not subjects made no response when the buzzer went off. Nonetheless, when questioned the next morning the majority of testees insisted that they had not slept a wink all night, thereby demonstrating that their sleeplessness was to some degree imagined.

How can an MS patient determine the specific cause of his or her sleep problems? In general, certain kinds of sleep disturbances have recurrent patterns associated with them. The insomnia caused by depression, for example, usually takes the following two forms:

1. A person will fall asleep in the evening with relatively little trouble. Several hours later he or she will wake up and find it almost impossible to get back to sleep for the rest of the night.

2. A person will fall asleep easily, then wake up like clockwork several hours later, usually around three or four o'clock. From this point on the rest of the night will be spent tossing and turning, with the person enjoying a kind of occasional semidoze at best.

Both these patterns are typical of depression as opposed to difficulty *getting* to sleep, general restlessness, and light sleep, all of which more often result from inactivity during the day.

Two other forms of sleep problems, both easy to diagnose, are caused by spasticity and weak bladder. In the first case, demyelinating disease in the spinal cord makes some patients prone to nocturnal spasticity, especially in the lower limbs. These spasms tend to come on suddenly, waking the victim violently—and painfully—from a sound sleep. Small doses of Valium or Xanax at bedtime will usually nip the problem in the bud. With sleep difficulties caused by urinary frequency, patients are advised to 1) cut down on their liquid intake at night; 2) void immediately before going to bed; 3) take appropriate medication as needed.

As an adjunct to these aids, be especially careful of caffeine drinks such as sodas, coffee, and tea. Coffee is a diuretic as well as a stimulant and must be used with care. If you drink it at all, drink it in the morning. Patients can also try warm milk with honey, or a calming herb tea such as chamomile or hops, both of which have been used as natural sedatives for centuries. Calcium supplements have proven helpful for some sleepless MS persons, and should be taken immediately before bed, as the body processes calcium most actively during the hours of sleep.

Tend also to the small things that cause subliminal discomfort: blankets that scratch, mattresses that sag, uncomfortable pillows, annoying room noises, poor ventilation, bad odors, blinking lights. And don't underestimate sleeping late in the mornings as a cause of insomnia. Many persons have found that simply getting up an hour or two earlier in the morning has allowed them to sleep better—and stay asleep—at night. Beware also of long afternoon naps. They use up our slumber chits, as it were, and throw the body's inner sleep clock out of sync.

What about sleeping pills? They are useful for occasional

bouts of sleeplessness. But as you know, overuse will cause addiction. Before turning to the stronger prescription sedatives, why not try over-the-counter brands first such as Nytol or Sominex. For some people their relatively gentle sleep-inducing effects are enough to push one over the fine line between wakefulness and sleep. If these don't work, an occasional dose of a standard sleep medication such as doxipen (trade name Sinequan) used in small doses of 10 or 20 mgs will almost always do the trick.

Finally, there is mental relaxation. Tension, discomfort, and a low-lying anxiety are often at the bottom of sleeplessness in MS patients, and one of the better means of addressing them is through presleep body relaxation. The following method, used today in many European hospitals and institutions, is designed to detense the entire body and prepare the mind for sleep. Try it.

1. Lie on your back with your arms at your sides and your legs comfortably extended.

2. Take several deep breaths. Relax as thoroughly as possible.

3. Start by concentrating on the top of your head. Tense the muscles of your scalp as tightly as possible and hold the tension for approximately five seconds. Then release. Feel the looseness and relaxation that result. Next, tense your forehead, hold, release, relax. Now the eyes. The nose (flare the nostrils and tighten the entire nose). The mouth. The ears, the back of the head, the chin. Feel the reflex loosening effect that follows after tightening each muscle group.

4. Proceed in this way slowly and systematically down the entire body. The neck should be tightened, then released and relaxed. Likewise the shoulders, chest, upper arms, lower arms, wrists, hands, rib cage, abdomen, upper and lower back, hips, buttocks, groin, thighs, knees, calves, ankles, feet, and toes.

5. While practicing the tension and relaxation exercise, make certain that your mind remains passive. Avoid worry and preoccupation. Keep your concentration centered on the muscle groups that are being tightened; or dwell on pleasant thoughts. Disturbing mental imagery of any kind is counterproductive to relaxation, and should be avoided.

6. When the exercise is completed—it should take around five minutes—draw several deep breaths and relax even more. Repeat this exercise several times if needed.

Here are other suggestions from MS patients who have coped with sleep difficulties:

Ida M.: I find that when my leg gets twitching and burning at night and if I can't sleep I try tightening it several times in a row, and putting ice packs on it. That usually calms it down. The coolness of the ice pack helps me relax myself entirely.

Donald: Sometimes I have trouble sleeping, sometimes I don't. I take a glass of warm lemon juice with honey at night, every night, and a single aspirin. They calm me down when I'm jittery or restless. I'll also take calcium pills with magnesium in it for sleep which my girlfriend recommended. She also has MS and says it works for her.

Sue E.: I'm up and down a hundred times each night going to the bathroom, so it drives me crazy. The trouble is that I can be sleeping, my bladder wakes me up, I'll walk out into the hall to go to the bathroom, and by the time I get back to bed all this activity has woken me up. I now keep one of those plastic urinals with a handle close to the bed every night so I can just use it there and not wake myself up walking around so much.

Ernest: I get woken up at night sometimes with pains in my legs and stiffness. I take my Lioresal and just turn over and go back to sleep. Sometimes it works, sometimes it doesn't.

Bill K.: Ordinary nonprescription sleeping pills always do the trick when I use them. My mind is buzzing at night and my body feels tired out and unhappy—it's hard to explain. But I can't get to sleep. These pills do it for me. The problem with them is that I've noticed if you take them too much they lose their effectiveness. So I lay off them for a couple of weeks at a time and then go back, and they work okay for a while longer.

COPING WITH TENSION AND STRESS

The ordinary stress of life is difficult enough. Couple it with the tension caused by MS discomfort and patients often find themselves tied into double knots.

Mild tranquilizers such as Valium are always an option, and some patients use them already as a spasticity relaxer. A small dose—one-quarter part of a 2-milligram pill, for instance—is a very effective relaxant.

Tranquilizer dependence is generally not a desirable condition for several reasons, however, not the least of which is the drowsiness and side effects, plus the fact that Valium and other benzodiazepine tranquilizers can cause debilitating leg weakness. Patients are advised to try milder alternatives first and turn to antitension medication only as a last resort.

Over the past years many specifics have been put forward for this enduring problem. Several of the better ones are as follows:

Relaxation Exercises

Here are two excellent methods for inducing relaxation:

1. Find a quiet place away from all distractions. Sit silently for a minute or two, then close your eyes. Let your muscles unwind. Take several deep breaths.

Imagine that your body is filled with water (i.e., tension) and that you intend to drain the water out through imaginary holes in your hands and feet. Start at the top of your head. Make a mental image of the water level as it slowly drains down from your forehead, down past your eyes, your nose, your chin, neck, shoulders. Drain the water down each arm and out the fingers. Picture the water level dropping to your chest, stomach, groin, thighs, calves, and then flowing out through the imaginary holes in the bottoms of your feet. Picture yourself totally empty and utterly relaxed.

Repeat this process several times. Notice that certain areas that you detensed just a moment ago have tightened up already. Relax them again. At each repetition you will feel increasingly unwound.

2. The second exercise is a mild form of self-hypnosis. For some persons it proves highly effective.

Sit comfortably, relax for several minutes, and take three or four deep breaths. Now mentally repeat the following suggestions to yourself, more or less to this effect: "My eyelids are getting heavy. They are starting to close, starting to feel as if lead weights were attached to them. I am becoming more and more tired, heavy, relaxed, so relaxed. I am feeling drowsy. It's getting harder and harder to keep my eyes open. My lids are getting heavier and heavier, and now my eyes are beginning to blink. I will let them blink. This is a sign that they are getting ready to close. They want to close. I will let them close. They are closing. Slowly and steadily. I am becoming more and more relaxed. I am sinking into a blissful, relaxed state. It's so hard to keep my eyes open now as I become more relaxed, more at ease, more heavy and relaxed. Harder and harder to keep them open. I'm sinking into a deep, relaxed state. More and more and more."

The first time you perform this exercise you may be surprised to see that your eyes *are* in fact closing. It is always something of a shock to find out how responsive we are to self-suggestion. Repeat these self-hypnotic phrases until your eyes close firmly. The process shouldn't take more than a few minutes.

Once your eyes are shut, continue to give yourself antistress suggestions in more or less the following terms. You are now going to deepen what has already become a light self-hypnotic trance: "Now that my eyes are closed, I am sinking more and more into a deep, quiet state where nothing in the world can hurt or bother me or cause me pain. I am totally at peace. I am sinking deeper and deeper, totally relaxed and absorbed. Outside noises and disturbances do not affect me in the slightest way. I feel so drowsy, so comfortable, so happy. I am relaxing more and more, sinking more and more with every breath I take. My whole body feels as if it has turned to lead. The outside world is disappearing. Every part of my body is relaxed now. My arms . . . my hands . . . my neck . . . the back of my head . . . my chest . . . my stomach . . . my knees . . . my feet . . . everything. I feel as if I am sinking into the chair (or bed), getting heavier and heavier. So relaxed now. I could move if I want to, but I don't because I am too comfortable and relaxed. My arms are pleasantly heavy. My legs. My head. All so comfortably relaxed. Nothing bothers me now. The deeper I go the more pleasant and relaxed I feel. I am getting heavier and heavier, sinking with a pleasant sense of weight. I am letting go. Deeper and deeper and deeper."

If this exercise is done properly, you should by now be in a pleasant, floating state, alert yet divorced from the outside world and to a certain extent from the body itself. The whole process so far should require about five to ten minutes to take effect. Remain in this state of relaxation and contentment for several minutes. When you are ready to quit, tell yourself that you wish to end the session, that you will emerge from it feeling refreshed and serene, ready to go about your business of the day feeling worry-free and rested. Take about a minute to give yourself these instructions. This last part is important and should not be skipped.

Practice this exercise daily, preferably at the same time each day. A good help is to prerecord your monologue on a cassette tape and play it back to yourself at each session. This trick allows you to stay entirely relaxed during the process without having to make even the mental effort of talking to yourself.

Biofeedback

Many physiological functions such as circulation, pulse, skin temperature, and blood pressure work without the mind's conscious participation. Recent developments in biological electronics have addressed this situation and created mechanical devices that help us gain some measure of control over these functions. The biofeedback machine is perhaps the best known.

Clinical biofeedback is ordinarily done on an electromyograph (EMG) machine, using electrodes attached to the person's forehead to monitor muscle changes. These changes are registered by a series of high-pitched sounds (or sometimes flashes of light, beeps, etc.) that rise and fall in synchronization with shifting tensions. This method of continuous monitoring creates a precise graph of the patient's muscular activity as the muscles grow alternately more and less relaxed.

While monitoring the sounds of the machine, the patient and the biofeedback therapist work together on a set of visualization and relaxation exercises. As relaxation increases, the machine emits sounds at increasingly lower frequencies. This information creates a feedback loop within the patient's mind, reinforcing his or her determination to continue relaxing plus an increased sensitivity to the body's subtle physiological processes.

Eventually, by regular use of biofeedback, patients learn to gain a degree of control over their normally automatic physiological processes. The final goal is to become free of the machine entirely and to manipulate these body functions by the power of mind alone. Home biofeedback machines, though less sophisticated than those used in clinics, are available from many medical suppliers and have helped many thousands of people to work against stress.

Physical Exercise

The subject of exercise has been thoroughly covered in a previous chapter. Here it should simply be mentioned that a daily regime of exercise suited to the MS person's needs and endurance level is an excellent specific against stress and should be put to use on a day-to-day basis if possible.

The exercise systems outlined in the above chapter are all useful in this regard. So are yoga; low-impact, nonendurance sports such as walking, canoeing, rowing, swimming; work on exercise equipment adapted to the patient's needs; and any other activity that stimulates the heart, quickens circulation, increases muscle tone, brings oxygen to the cells, and works against the nervousness that so often results from prolonged periods of inactivity. The body is meant to be active; to the best of your ability, keep it that way.

PAY ATTENTION TO YOUR PSYCHOLOGICAL NEEDS

To the best of your ability, get organized. Postponed phone calls, letters not written, obligations not met, untidy environments, all can have a subliminal but very real stressful impact on a person's day. Keep checklists, calendars, schedules. Start the morning by reviewing your day's obligations, and then methodically measure your time and the energy quota you have to fulfill them. Know your limits. Choose your priorities carefully and don't take on more work than you can handle—nothing causes stress more quickly than an overloaded schedule. Guard against procrastination. Don't be afraid to say no.

When you feel the urge, cry. Crying is a great way to relieve anxiety and reduce psychological strain. When we hold back tears we hold back tension too.

Avoid setting difficult or impossible goals and then scolding yourself when you don't get them done. Such behavior is guaranteed to cause stress. Educators have shown us time and time again that the best way to approach any task is by planned, measured increments. If you have a job to accomplish, plan on doing the first two steps today, the next two steps tomorrow, then finish up the day after. In other words, set manageable goals and stick to them. If they prove unmanageable, revise them until they work for you. A step at a time is always better than one fell swoop. The National Multiple Sclerosis Society's helpful pamphlet *Coping with Stress* has much to say on this subject, and it's free for the asking. A useful sample:

> When you usually have limited energy, it's natural to work harder on days you feel well. Instead of getting worn out trying to do everything, organize each day the night before or in the morning.

Plan to do the most stressful or difficult task early in the day.

Schedule rest periods, and remember to take them before you get worn out.

Pace your activities by doing a heavy task and then some light ones. Don't try to do too many heavy chores in one day.

Combine chores or errands so you can get more done with less effort.*

Watch your health. Stress and depression can be traced back to physical malaise as much as to the circumstances of life. Consult the prior chapters on exercise and health maintenance.

Find a quiet place and visit it frequently. Tests have shown that stress levels are dramatically reduced when a person regularly schedules time off from the activities of life to calm down and let go for a few minutes of every day.

Share your problems. Suffering from symptoms of stress does not mean you are "troubled" or "different." It means you are human like the rest of us, and are in need of good advice or a shoulder to cry on. Don't neglect the value of family and good friends to help you through when the going gets rough. When life seems unmanageable, perhaps it's time to seek professional advice, or at least to talk to other MS patients who have experienced similar difficulties. Talking helps.

Finally, consider the cultivation of spiritual practice as a method for filling your psychological needs. Time and again health care professionals have witnessed that MS persons who are committed to something higher—be this a religious belief, a meditation practice, or a simple unselfish interest in service and placing other's needs before their own—are often those who thrive best, the ones who seem to remain most healthy, most active, most content. As many recovering addicts in twelve-step programs across the country now realize, meditation, prayer, and the belief in a higher power serve as anchors, keeping a person centered and confident, even in the midst of life's most ferocious storms.

*Coping with Stress, National Multiple Sclerosis Society, adapted from an article in The Development Team, published by the Arthritis Foundation, 1314 Spring Street NW, Atlanta, Georgia, 1988.

If you have any inclination along these lines—or if you have left the church or denomination of your childhood and now feel a psychic void in its place—consider turning back to worship as a kind of emotional first aid for the problems that MS brings. If you have hesitations along these lines, simply keep the thought in mind, ponder on it from time to time, weigh the alternatives— and then remember the inscription written above the tomb of the famous Persian poet and saint, Jalalu'ddin Rumi. "Come back, come back!" the inscription reads, "there is still time!"

8

Special Concerns in MS

Like any chronic disease, multiple sclerosis presents a series of challenges that are specific, if not unique, to the individuals who experience them. Certain of these challenges are physical; certain ones psychological; most are a combination of both. All are typical of MS, and all can be coped with if the knowledge and resources are in place.

In this chapter we will have a look at the most important of these challenges and discover what can be done to make them negotiable in the course of everyday living.

DEALING WITH MS ON THE JOB

There are several troublesome quandaries that tend to arise for MS persons who work at a steady or part-time job.

The first is perhaps the most widely discussed among MS patients: disclosure. Should MS persons tell their employers and coworkers that they have multiple sclerosis?

To begin, some people feel there is a moral imperative involved in this issue, that it is a matter of ethical correctness to be forthright with one's work associates and with one's present (or potential) employers over this key matter. Especially if the MS person is in the process of seeking a job and going through the usual interview procedures, there may be internal pressure to get things out in the open from the start, and to hedge one's bets, as it were, by warning people in advance.

Is disclosure necessary? Should one tell?

Let's answer this question by first setting the record straight: a person suffering from MS, or from any other visible or invisible disability, has no *legal obligation* to inform others, either employer or coworkers, about his or her condition. It is by no means against the law to withhold this information.

That said, the moral question remains: Is it ethically dishonest not to tell?

The answer, as with many moral dilemmas, is that it depends on personal choice. If you feel compelled to tell, then tell. If not, remain silent. It's up to you.

On the pro side is the fact that disclosure gets one's cards out on the table from the beginning. This line of action relieves persons of concern that their condition will inadvertently be "discovered," and that they will lose their jobs as a result, not only because they have the disease but because they "lied" during the job interview. On the con side are the facts that MS persons may not be hired in the first place if they tell. Or they will be given less responsible positions within the organization, and here will be looked upon by employers and co-workers alike as "special cases" deserving of that strange combination so many MS people experience of cloying solicitation and patronizing disregard.

Whatever course you decide to take, realize that many MS persons have made a point of being honest during job interviews, only to find the doors of employment slammed in their face. Indeed, the sorry fact is that hiring agents are often consciously or unconsciously biased against people with handicaps, and that they frequently choose applicants not as well qualified as the MS candidate purely out of ignorance and misplaced concern.

Again, it's your choice. Think the matter over carefully, knowing that you are under no obligations other than those you impose upon yourself. Indeed, having seen the prejudicial treatment others receive in the workplace, many MS patients today opt to remain silent during the initial job interview, and later on, once they have proved their value at work, to quietly and carefully inform employers and coworkers about their condition. As Marianne Rose, Director of Operation Job Match in the National Capital Chapter of the National Multiple Sclerosis Society, went on record as saying several years ago vis-à-vis the disclosure issue, "Our policy is, this is a decision you have to make for yourself."*

If and when a person decides to disclose the facts, what is the best way to go about it? The following points, adapted from advice garnered from the Job Raising program of the National Multiple Sclerosis Society, are all worth considering:

• Be careful of disclosing your condition too early during the course of employment. Get secure in your job first and prove your value. Then tell.

• When you talk about your MS, don't make the disclosure overly dramatic. Speak of it in concrete terms and be careful not to volunteer unnecessary details, either about your physical problems or your emotional response to the symptoms. Answer questions in concise terms, without raising issues you'd rather not discuss. "I made the mistake when I was interviewing for a job," one MS patient reports, "of complaining about my vision problems to my boss. When I did this she got very flustered and started to ask what would happen if I hurt myself moving around the office, and might the company be held liable? She was concerned whether I was able to read the fine print in some of our documents, whether or not I'd make this mistake or that mistake. None of this would have happened if I hadn't been so specific about my seeing problems in the first place, and if I had answered her questions in general terms without going into the details."

Rule of thumb: If they don't ask, don't tell them.

*National Multiple Sclerosis Society Facts & Issues Newsletter, June 1989.

• Be prepared ahead of time. Some experts suggest that MS persons write down what they intend to discuss during disclosure, and rehearse the scenario mentally or with others. This way a patient's presentation will be clear and unconfused, and a sense of confidence will pervade the dialogue.

• Be self-assured, forthright, and nondefensive. Avoid arguing or self-justification—you are simply reporting the facts. If questions of your competency arise, point out that you are doing an adequate job so far, and that you intend to keep it this way. Avoid appealing to a person's sympathies or pity. Present yourself as just another hard worker, a concerned employee who happens to have a certain physical problem, which is manageable and which does not interfere in any significant way with your ability to get the job done.

All in all, if a boss or supervisor sees that an MS person is secure in his or her ability to deal with the disease, if the patient seems legitimately concerned with the situation but not obsessed, and if a satisfactory performance is being turned in during work hours, chances are strong that others will understand and be supportive.

• Some patients are concerned about fatigue in the workplace. We know that this problem is common to many MS persons, and that it can slow a person down at the most inappropriate moments. When it does, the patient may feel an overwhelming need to rest and to get away for a few minutes. But this impulse will not always be looked on in a kindly light by one's boss and coworkers. What to do?

Although there are always notable exceptions, most coworkers are tolerant about such things, and many will respect a patient's courage for coping as well as he or she does. Often it's simply a matter of conditioning others to the fact that one has these weak spells, and that now and then a rest is needed. The bottom line, after all, is how well one has performed on the job at the end of the day and the end of the month. When this contribution is substantial, a few minutes taken off now and then will seem inconsequential.

At certain times, of course, one's fatigue will be overwhelming, and MS persons may have to excuse themselves for the day. This is often an embarrassing and worrisome situation, but sometimes it cannot be helped. The fact of the matter is that on certain days functioning is difficult, and one's coworkers will just have to understand. A few extra days off now and then, or a half-day lost here and there may result. It is simply the way it is. It is the reality of the situation.

Finally, if at any point it becomes too difficult to remain at one's job, other options always remain open. Due to advancements in communications and computer-based technology, we are entering a golden age of home employment, and more opportunities for home-based jobs exist today than ever before.

MS persons will, for example, find that a number of accredited professional, vocational, and college courses can be studied by mail correspondence. Vocational training for home-based businesses is readily available, and numbers of money-making opportunities can be pursued in one's own living room or basement, with oneself as boss. Associations such as the National Vocational Guidance Association (1607 New Hampshire Avenue N.W., Washington, DC 20009), the American Personnel and Guidance Association (1607 New Hampshire Avenue N.W., Washington, DC 20009), the American Rehabilitation Counseling Association (1607 New Hampshire Avenue N.W., Washington, DC 20009), and the B'nai B'rith Career and Counseling Services (1640 Rhode Island Avenue N.W., Washington, DC 20009) will all provide literature, referrals, and advice concerning home-based employment.

If you need to find out more, the following pamphlets are all worth sending for:

Tips on Home Study Schools
National Home Study Council
1601 Eighteenth Street N.W.
Washington, DC 20009

Three Steps for College Entrance
President's Committee on Employment of the Handicapped
Washington, DC 20210

Guide to Independent Study Through Correspondence Instructions
National University Extension Associates
One Dupont Circle
Suite 360
Washington, DC 20036

Directory of Accredited Home Study Schools
National Home Study Council
1601 Eighteenth Street N.W.
Washington, DC 20009

Student Aids in the Space Age: Education Resources for the Handicapped
B'nai B'rith Career and Counseling Services
1640 Rhode Island Avenue N.W.
Washington, DC 20036

PREGNANCY AND PARENTING: THE CHOICE IS YOURS

Although for many years it was thought that pregnancy in some way encouraged MS flareups, today it is believed by many doctors that pregnancy actually exerts a temporary protective influence *against* exacerbation, that it in no way worsens the prospect of future disabilities occurring with MS, and that, all in all, a woman with multiple sclerosis can look forward to bearing children with approximately the same degree of risk as any healthy mother.

At the same time, having children is a full-time, labor-intensive job, as any parent will agree, and one that drains enormous amounts of a parent's patience, time, and energy. A young woman with MS already suffering from fatigue and other disabilities may suddenly find herself with a needful infant on her hands and not enough strength to provide adequate care. The decision for a woman with MS as to whether or not to have a child is thus based not on the question "Can I?" but "Should I?"

This question poses enormous implications, and the answer

that a husband and wife arrive at together will have repercussions of one kind or another for the rest of their lives. Such a decision requires a major amount of thought and planning before it is reached. The following points of advice will help perspective parents focus their questions on this difficult issue, and help them assess the potential pluses and minuses that are involved in an MS parenthood.

1. *Make as thorough and honest an assessment of your present condition as possible.*

Whether or not you and your spouse decide to have a child should depend to a large extent on your prognosis.

For example, if you are symptom free, and if you have been this way for some time, having a child is clearly a feasible option.

If, on the other hand, you seem to be on a relapsing-progressive trajectory, and if your physician believes that the prognosis is likely to continue in this direction and even become more severe as time passes, then a great deal of serious reflection must be given to the prospect of having a child—both for your own sake and for the sake of the child.

To get clear on this matter, a thorough and entirely honest physical self-appraisal is necessary early in the game. In the long run, only you can know what it is like to live inside your body; and only you can assess just how much energy and wherewithal you really have for the demanding job of raising a child.

Do be careful not to hedge on this one; face the facts as squarely and courageously as you can. And while you're pondering the matter, take your time. Chances are that no one is pressuring you, and you owe it to yourself to consider the realities as prudently and thoughtfully as possible.

2. *Know the risks beforehand.*

As part of the self-assessment process it is valuable to be aware of the specific physical difficulties you may run into as a parent, and to consider them accordingly in terms of your own situation. Some possible examples include:

• Do you experience consistent bouts of undue fatigue? Are they getting better? Worse? More frequent? More incapacitating?

• Do you take strong medications some or much of the time? Certain of these preparations, such as ACTH, other steroids, and immunosuppressants, are counterindicated during pregnancy.

• Do you have major gait and balance disturbances that might interfere with your ability to carry safely or with your ability to transfer a child from place to place?

• Are your relapses becoming more frequent and more severe?

• Is your eyesight strong enough to keep close watch on a toddler during the danger years of two through five?

• Do you have trouble using your hands or holding on to things? Might weakness and lack of coordination affect your ability to pick up a baby and handle it correctly?

• Are you wheelchair-bound—or does your prognosis indicate that you soon will be?

It's really a matter of degree. If you suffer one or more of the difficulties listed above, but if they are infrequent and not severe, then perhaps they will not pose a major problem. If they are severe, this is serious food for thought.

When assessing risk potential mothers should also know that during the six months following birth they will be especially prone to flareups and to such postpartum problems as anemia, fatigue, stress, and infection. An article in *Inside MS* magazine adds the following caveats:

> In practical terms, adequate rest, treatment of anemia, minimizing stress, and avoiding infection and temperature elevation may all contribute to reducing the risk of postpartum relapse. In the U.S., many women on maternity leave must return to work six to eight weeks after delivery. Since this coincides with the period of high risk for relapse, it should be considered carefully before a pregnancy is attempted, especially if the patient's employer has not been told that she had the disease.*

*Inside MS, Spring 1992.

3. *Make it a joint decision.*

In a family where one of the spouses has MS, spouses have a tendency to place the burden of decision entirely on the person with the disease. But this approach can end up causing resentments on both sides later on. As with marriage, parenthood is a mutual affair, and both parties will be forced to make sizable accommodations when the child arrives. Husband and wife should therefore participate equally in the decision-making process, and both should be clear concerning the sacrifices and adjustments that will be demanded. Healthy spouses would do well to ask themselves the following questions:

- Am I willing to spend time—possibly a great deal of time— providing child care when and if my spouse goes into relapse, or when he or she is feeling out of sorts?

- Am I willing to spend time and energy learning the new skills that child care demands?

- If my spouse's energy is limited, am I willing to take up the slack by doing the jobs that he or she was once responsible for, such as household chores, yard duties, driving family members, taking care of an older parent, shopping for food, doing laundry, and so forth?

- Will I be able to deal with the added tension and stress that having children brings?

- If circumstances force me to work only part time and to spend the remainder of the day taking care of the child, will we survive financially?

- If my spouse becomes entirely incapacitated owing to relapse or a worsening of the MS condition, am I willing to become the primary caregiver for the child? If so, do I have the endurance, know-how, and time to do it all?

- Do my professional and life circumstances allow me to take enough time off at home for parenting? Will I find myself burdened to the point of overload if I take on the tasks of earning a living *and* of caring for a child?

• In case my spouse's condition becomes particularly severe, am I willing—and capable—of taking care of both the child *and* the sick spouse?

Hard questions. Very hard. While the answers can only be estimates at best, and while there are no rights or wrongs, the emotional implications that surround these issues and the fact that there are no canned answers to any of them, in a sense makes it even more difficult to see the picture clearly and to reach final conclusions.

At the same time, these questions relate to real-life matters that cannot be avoided and that must be seriously thought out before an informed decision is made. Again, take your time and weigh things in the balance. If you feel confused or intimidated by such choices, don't hesitate to seek advice, either from friends, family members, clergy, or professional counselors. Remember, what you decide now will influence your life for many years to come, and it is well worth taking the time and trouble to become clear before you act.

Finally, a common concern directly related to the above issues is whether or not MS spouses, be they husband or wife, are willing to relinquish at least some of the attention they are normally accustomed to receiving from the well mate. For, make no mistake about it, once a child enters the home well spouses will be forced to withdraw at least some of their attention from the MS person and direct it fully on the infant.

This modification of marital habit can be tough medicine for a man or woman who is used to being attended to without competition, and it must be considered an important part of the child-rearing picture. Ask yourself and your mate: How much do we really want a child? Do the benefits outweigh the risks? How much are we willing to give up—and what kinds of lifestyle changes and pressures are we willing to assume—to have one?

Then act accordingly.

4. *Determine your resources.*

From the day the child enters the house MS parents will need all the help they can get.

During the postpartum period, for instance, exacerbations tend to increase severalfold, most likely because of the pressures and stress of having a new child in the house. What kinds of assistance will be on hand if and when flareups occur? How much help will the well spouse be able to contribute during this time? Will you be financially able to hire a mother's aide or an outside assistant? Are family members and friends available?

It is wise policy, in other words, to take inventory of your potential support lines now, while in the planning stage, and to organize them in advance of the birth. Knowing that help exists is a help in itself.

If, in fact, it appears that you are lacking in childrearing help, now is the time to do something about it. Seek advice from friends and doctors and community-assistance organizations. Talk to other MS parents. Discuss matters with your parents, and with your spouse. Talk to occupational therapists about setting up your household so that it makes child care easier and more efficient. They are experts in the field of home adaptation and will have much useful advice to contribute that you probably wouldn't think of on your own. Certain obstetricians specialize in dealing with MS births. Seek them out and get their guidance.

Potential sources of help include:

- The well spouse
- Physicians and medical health-care professionals
- Occupational therapists
- Medical referral services
- Parents and grandparents
- Brothers and sisters
- Aunts, uncles, cousins, etc.
- Older children
- Mother's aides
- Community parental-help organizations

5. *Talk to other MS parents.*

Go directly to the horse's mouth: talk to other MS parents who have gone the child-care route and who know the score. See how they have handled specific problems. Ask for tips, shortcuts, guidance on matters that you are particularly concerned with. Attend MS groups. Members here are a treasure trove of down-to-earth, hands-on information, not only about child raising but about contingent matters that you may not yet anticipate. And if members are not able to answer questions they will usually know who can. Do, however, act early. Well informed is well prepared.

MAKING SEX WORK

Sexual performance, that most personal and tender matter, is a concern that impacts on almost all MS patients, sometimes in a palpable physical way, sometimes via the turbulent emotions that sexual change brings about. The first question most MS persons therefore ask themselves is: In what ways—if any—will this disease alter my ability to have, and enjoy, sexual relations?

As usual, there are no definitive answers. An individual with a mild case of MS, or a case that has remained asymptomatic for long periods of time, probably has few worries in this area. Of greater concern is when the relapsing-remitting variety of the disease predominates, and even more so when a case of MS is rapidly progressive. Persons afflicted in these ways commonly experience sexual disorders, though the degree of involvement varies widely from patient to patient. In general, men tend to be affected more than women, though statistically speaking patients of both sexes are likely to develop some kind of physical or emotional difficulty during the course of their illness, especially if they suffer from bladder disorders.

A brief inventory of the physio-sexual malfunctions that may occur from MS includes the following: decrease of sensation in the vagina or penis; premature, delayed, or absent ejaculation and loss of the pleasurable sensations it produces; slowed sexual responsiveness and arousal time; painful orgasm; permanent or intermittent inability to attain erection; weakness or spasticity of the pelvic muscles; vaginal dryness; genital pain and discomfort.

Also to be considered are the effects that muscle spasms, bladder disorders, tremor, fatigue, and pain have on sexual performance. Some MS patients, moreover, experience no specific sexual deficits, yet report an overall decrease in erotic energy and concern. Finally, as if this list is not long enough, the emotional fluctuations MS persons go through over sexual loss are often as devastating as the dysfunctions themselves.

For example, newly diagnosed patients often begin to think of themselves as ugly and undesirable. Many are very young and have had a minimal amount of dating experience. Influenced by the pervasive outlook of the youth culture, which emphasizes the importance of appearance alone, they have not yet learned that there is more to attraction than physical looks, and that a really satisfactory relationship is built on intimacy, shared interests, rapport, and commitment, as well as on sexual allure.

Such persons start thinking of themselves as "freaks," whose physical disabilities, they believe, will now discourage overtures of any kind from members of the opposite sex. Self-esteem and body image plummet. With them go all attempts to appear appealing and available. Who would want me now? persons ask themselves, and then act out their negative assumptions by withdrawing from the dating scene, often, ironically, before their fears have been borne out by experience. Even patients with no visible symptoms may think of themselves as harboring a "dirty little secret" that if discovered will automatically put an end to any intimate relationship. Why try in the first place with such a handicap? they ask themselves, thus launching a self-fulfilling prophesy.

A husband or wife with MS may feel awkward and unattractive to a spouse when unclothed and in bed. Is my husband, my wife, staying with me out of pity, patients ask themselves, now that I wear a catheter so much of the day, and my body is so unattractive? Doesn't the fact that I have to interrupt a lovemaking session to go to the bathroom, or that my leg cramps up in the middle of the act, or that my movements during lovemaking are so jerky, seem bizarre and distasteful to my spouse? Hasn't my body become a turnoff? Wouldn't we be better off apart? Or at least in separate bedrooms?

These internal dialogues go on and on, with patients often selling themselves—and others—short by such dismal and often unnecessary fears.

What can be done to help? The following suggestions are based both on the experience of patients and on the counsel of professionals in the field.

1. *Communicate.*

The initial and perhaps most important step a couple can take to overcome—or at least to cope with—the sexual problems caused by MS is to *talk about them.* Utter silence between sexual partners is a dangerous game; indeed, unless husband and wife, boyfriend and girlfriend spell out for one another what it is they are thinking and feeling along these lines, the sexual life they share will soon become clouded with doubts, silent accusals, and unresolved imaginings.

This does not mean, of course, that couples must share every nuance of their inner psychic world; and certainly tact can be the wisest course at times. On the other hand, to refrain from discussing such critical issues as the physical changes that are affecting your sexual relationship, and the types of arousal techniques that work best for both parties is to court the misunderstandings that almost inevitably result from closed channels of communication. When in doubt, when in need, when in the dark—talk about it. Helen S., an MS patient, and her husband, Steve, discuss the importance of keeping the lines of discussion open and humming:

HELEN: At first I was real scared. Of myself mostly, not of Steve. I mean, I thought now that I had MS and was so much slower and more kind of lackadaisical he would lose interest in me sexually. So I just sort of shut down.

STEVE (LAUGHING): Yeah, and instead of telling me about it she kept giving me the slip at night! I started thinking I had B.O.!

HELEN: It was my fault. He was an angel, but I couldn't face talking about it and—what I thought would be—all the negative things he would say about how our sex life was over and lousy now. He finally sat me down and *made* me talk about it.

STEVE: It helped, didn't it?

HELEN: Yep. Sure did.

STEVE: She was unhappy about being frank with me when we first started to talk about sex, but I assured her—I told her I found her more attractive now than ever—kind of more vulnerable and sweet or something—and that we would work out all the sexual stuff slowly, together. Over time. I was in her corner, I told her.

HELEN: Oh, that made such a difference! Just hearing him say those things. I was so scared up to that time. The worst thing I was doing was keeping it all bottled up inside me. As soon as it hit the light of day things got better for me. We've been able to really talk about it now, and to experiment. Some things definitely help.

Here are a few tips for enhancing communication on the subject of sex:

• Don't be afraid to spell out to your partner what it is that turns you on sexually and how he or she can go about doing it. Be as explicit as your relationship allows. The more information a mate has concerning an MS person's sexual needs, the more he or she can do to improve the interaction. Ignorance in this department is definitely not bliss.

• Patients should be frank and honest about their needs. At the same time, well mates should not be made to think that they carry the entire burden of arousal on their shoulders and that unless they perform with mechanical and emotional perfection the patient will be unfulfilled. Approach this issue from a "we" standpoint. Both partners are now working together, cooperating, not only to maximize the patient's sexuality but to enhance the pleasure of the well mate as well.

• If you are peeved at your mate for a sexual blunder or for being insensitive to your physical needs, avoid angry accusations. Avoid all "you" messages, all extreme adverbs such as "always" and "never." These terms will simply arouse similar anger and hurt on the partner's end.

Instead, choose your words carefully, emphasizing your feelings rather than the partner's mistakes. For example:

Avoid: "You just aren't spending enough time getting me excited."

Better: "I sometimes feel we're not taking enough time together to get me aroused."

Avoid: "You never pay any attention to the things I ask you to do."

Better: "You're doing a great job getting me excited, but there are still some things you can do that would really help. Like for instance . . ."

Avoid: "Why do you never let me know when I'm hurting you?"

Better: "It would make me feel a lot better if you promised to tell me whenever I'm hurting you. That way I can avoid giving you pain."

Avoid: "You never talk about your sexual feelings with me."

Better: "I want to share more with you about the sexual problems we're having right now."

Avoid: "You hurt me when you come into me. My muscles get all tense and tight; you have to be more gentle and careful with me when we make love."

Better: "The muscles in my groin tend to tighten up and get uncomfortable when we make love. It's not your fault at all, of course, we just have to work out a better method together."

• Avoid discussing sensitive sexual matters when you are annoyed at your mate or when both of you are overtired. Wait until a more mellow mood prevails; then bring it up. If things are not going well during the actual lovemaking session, moreover, it is okay to make tactful suggestions; it is definitely *not* a smart idea to launch into a discussion at this sensitive moment or to interrupt the flow with a lengthy critical dissertation. Save this for later when you are both in the proper frame of mind.

2. *Explore your sexual options.*

If a person's sexuality is altered or diminished by neurological disease, this will probably mean that his or her ability to respond sexually is altered as well. It does *not* mean that this person can no longer enjoy sex, only that the path to enjoyment now lies along different and perhaps unexplored lines.

For example, if patients are no longer able to have orgasm during regular intercourse, masturbation may prove an effective substitute.

Women who have become vaginally dry will find an impressive array of vaginal lubricants and jellies offered for sale at any drugstore.

If the MS spouse experiences excessive fatigue during intercourse, partners are advised to choose their lovemaking times of day or night carefully. Note, for instance, that morning sex energy is usually stronger than afternoon, afternoon sex energy stronger than evening. Find the best time of day for maximum arousal and, if possible, plan your lovemaking sessions around it. Some physicians also suggest that patients rest for an hour or so before having intercourse. It's a good idea as well to have sex before eating, not after—a full stomach can make lovers logy and slow.

When a man has difficulty gaining or keeping an erection, he can still satisfy his mate by providing clitoral stimulation. He may also find that although he is unable to maintain an erection long enough to climax during intercourse, manual stimulation of his penis will produce a satisfying sexual experience. Mutual masturbation, in fact, is an alternative sexual technique that has been successfully adopted by many couples.

Men who have difficulty achieving an erection may find that

manipulation of the penis in its flaccid state produces adequate pleasure. Note also that there are clinical options to consider. "If a man's erections are not sufficient for penetration or intercourse," claims a team of doctors writing on the management of sexual dysfunction, "surgically implanted prostheses may be an appropriate option. These include a rigid, noninflatable rod prosthesis and a semirigid inflatable device. Good results have also been obtained with the injection of papaverine, a drug that dilates blood vessels, directly into the penis just prior to intercourse."*

In some instances taking medication at the proper times will overcome sexual problems. Persons suffering from spasticity, for example, may find a dose of medication immediately before intercourse reduces their chances of spasms and of "locking up." "For women and men with MS," writes Dr. Michael Barrett, "adductor spasms of the thighs may make intercourse difficult. Some people cope with this by timing their antispasmodic medications for maximum effect at the time they are planning sexual activity . . . or they may position pillows to accommodate spasms should they occur."**

Patients who are slow to respond sexually may find that a change of scene, a new bed or bedroom in which to make love, sexy underwear or lingerie, scented body oil, an exciting sexual variation, a presex massage session, stimulating music, incense, perfumes and cologne, erotic talk during intercourse, a new position, a mutually shared sexual fantasy, a prolonged and attentive period of genital caressing will help in arousal.

Patients who experience decreased genital sensitivity may discover that erotic enhancers such as a manual vibrator or other sex aids help in the process of self-excitement. They may also find that by giving explicit directions to their mates concerning the best methods of arousal—or even by performing these manipulations on themselves at the appropriate moment—satisfaction can be more easily achieved.

Finally, it should be said that in some cases it may simply be

*Randall Schapiro, ed., *Symptom Management in Multiple Sclerosis*. New York, Demos Publications, 1987.

**Sexuality and Multiple Sclerosis*. New York, Multiple Sclerosis Society, 1976.

impossible for the MS person to climax properly and to achieve the usual pleasures that accompany a successful orgasm. When this occurs, patients often become despondent, believing that their sensuous life is over and that they will never again experience sexual satisfaction of any kind.

As many counselors and sex therapists have pointed out through the years, one of the principal causes of such thinking is so-called "goal-oriented sex"—that is, sex that has orgasm through intercourse as its single aim. When this approach is taken exclusively—and assuming that a patient has difficulty achieving climax—the outcome is often a no-win event for everybody involved.

There is, however, an alternative approach persons affected in this way can consider. Instead of assuming that the only pathway to sexual satisfaction is through the ultimate experience of orgasm, they change their way of thinking, realizing that touching, kissing, caressing, stroking, genital manipulation, and all the other acts that we think of as preliminaries to intercourse can in fact be made the very center of the sexual experience. "Society emphasizes 'normal' or 'proper' ways to obtain sexual gratification," we read in *Symptom Management in Multiple Sclerosis,* "which tends to make sex goal-oriented towards intercourse and orgasm. Many people find great physical and psychological satisfaction from those activities traditionally termed 'foreplay.' One excellent way to decrease or completely eliminate pressures and expectation is to become less goal-oriented by renaming such activities as 'sexplay.' Sexual expression may be directed to parts of the body other than the genitals, increasing cuddling, caressing, massage or other forms of touch, and it may involve experimenting with masturbation, vibrators, or other devices."*

Patients who experience difficulty achieving orgasm or who have become impotent should thus consider changing both their priorities and their sexual modus operandi. Instead of setting their sights exclusively on climax, they now restructure their lovemak-

---

*Randall Schapiro, ed., *Symptom Management in Multiple Sclerosis.* New York, Demos Publications, 1987.

ing technique, proceeding more slowly than before, taking time to caress and savor, becoming more sensuous and tactile, enjoying their mates' pleasure more and thinking less about their own orgasmic sensations. The session is then perhaps ended with a course of mutual masturbation or a variation on this theme.

A substitute, perhaps, but all in all not a bad one. Indeed, for many persons this approach opens up entirely new doors and comes surprisingly close to providing a complete and satisfying alternative to normal orgasm-oriented sex. For those so inclined, or so in need, it's worth a try.

3. *Have realistic expectations and set attainable goals.*

There is no doubt about it, in many cases MS will decrease one's ability to enjoy the game of sex. This is simply the way it is now. This is how things stand. The best thing one can do under the circumstances is to grieve for a time—and then get on with it.

Start by setting attainable goals and by readjusting expectations. The fact is that MS patients and their mates may be making love less frequently than before, or that their general level of arousal and capability will be reduced. Orgasm may be difficult to attain; muscular cramps and spasms become a part of life; things just aren't the same. To assume, therefore, that one's sex life will be exactly as it was before the MS arrived—or that one's sexual problems will someday magically go away on their own—is not realistic.

At the same time, one's glass is also half-full, and there are many options still open for attaining sexual satisfaction. Determine what these options are through experience and experiment, be honest with yourself about the conclusions, and act accordingly. A male MS patient gives us his insights on the question of expectations:

Sam S.: You can't believe it at first. What worked on your body before doesn't work as well now. I kept thinking, hell, the next time we make love I'll be able to get an erection like in the good old days. If I try hard enough. Just concentrate more and keep working out. My wife, Leslie, will get me going. But you know, it's an unpredictable thing now. So I live with it. Sometimes I get a good erection. Once in a while. I never know when it's coming, and I'm happy for it when it does. But I don't expect it. I expect that Leslie and I will do a lot of caressing, I'll stimulate her till she's happy, she'll work on me as best she can. That's what I expect. When it's better than that, well, hallelujah! If not, what can you do? You just cope, and get whatever enjoyment you can. All in all things could be a lot worse.

4. *Be aware of the effect medications have on your sexual performance.*

There are subtle variations on the sexual theme that MS patients and their mates sometimes overlook. One of these is the effect medications can have on sexual performance.

For example, patients who take Valium for spasticity may find themselves feeling listless and apathetic throughout the day; other tranquilizers and muscle relaxants produce the same effect. Antihistamines will make patients drowsy, and hence not inclined toward sex. The same is true for anticholinergic drugs such as Tofranil, which are frequently prescribed for MS-type bladder disorders. Antidepressants can interfere with male erection and with female lubrication. Symmetrel, given to combat fatigue, can produce jitteriness, dizziness, and mild depression, none of which are conducive to romance. And so on. A number of other pharmacological side effects may be experienced.

There are several steps you can take to improve the situation.

First, patients who are experiencing sexual dysfunction should discuss the matter with their doctors to determine if part of the problem is drug-related. If it is, a change of medication may be in order, or a reduction of dosage.

If it is not possible to change a medication, then patients should determine what time of day or night they prefer to have sex and set up their medication schedule to accommodate it. Occasionally, simply lowering the amount of a drug one has in their system at the time of making love is all that is necessary. Doctors will be happy to work with patients around this issue and to suggest alternative drug schedules. Sometimes this simple trick alone can go a long way toward correcting sexual difficulties.

5. *Plan ahead.*

Know your body, your habits, your disease, and your present limitations. Then plan ahead.

For example, nothing can take the romance out of love more quickly than a bout of incontinence during the sex act. So be prepared: Void your bladder before making love and go easy on liquids several hours before beginning. Some patients place a urinal, a bowl of water, and a washcloth by their bed when they are about to make love. Just in case the urge comes on suddenly, they have the facilities close at hand and can quickly return to their pleasures without undue interruption.

Another contingency to plan for is fatigue. We have already touched on this subject: patients are advised to get plenty of rest before sex, to pick their best times of day in advance, to make sure their medications do not cause drowsiness or lethargy, and to avoid eating until the act is completed. Some patients also find that coffee, soda, and other caffeine-containing drinks give them a presex pickup. For others—and this, of course, varies from person to person—a short bout of exercise before beginning gets the juices moving. Experiment.

For some MS persons, certain medications will help combat fatigue. If this is the case, take the drug shortly before beginning lovemaking. This simple act of preparation, in fact, is valuable for all symptoms of MS vis-à-vis sex; if a symptom is an impediment to lovemaking, be sure to take the appropriate medication for it *before* beginning.

Finally, patients should consider practicing a round or two of relaxation exercises before making love; the effects will be pleasant and beneficial for both partners, and in some cases it will beef up a patient's sexual stamina as well. See Chapter 7 for the details.

6. *If necessary, seek sexual counseling.*

In certain cases, especially when communication is poor between partners or when a patient suffers psychologically related sexual problems, a therapist or sex counselor may be consulted.

Therapists help in a number of ways. They may, for example, talk patients through their fears and self-doubts, supplying them with enough impartial advice to help them help themselves. Therapists serve as both mediator and arbitrator for sexually dysfunctional couples, pointing out the sexual games that each partner is playing, helping couples work through their psychic knots, providing advice for long-term and short-term interpersonal change. Finally, couples can share their problems with others like themselves in a group therapy setting. In many cases the group approach works wonders. Note:

Judith: Chuck and I had been married for two years when I developed MS. At first he was very willing to try and work things out with me, but when it became clear that I wasn't getting any better he started to withdraw from me, especially on a sexual level. I think he felt so overwhelmed and his only defense against the anger and frustration he was feeling was to retreat into his own little psychological world. This went on for about eight or nine months until I couldn't stand it anymore, and I begged him to come with me to group therapy. At first he was resistant, so I went on my own. I started coming back and telling him some of the things the therapist and other group members told me, and he was amazed, 'cause they seemed so accurate in their assessment of Chuck, even though they had never met him. After a while he started coming with me. He never regretted it. This group helped him see what he was doing. The therapist had a whole lot of advice to give us about how we could get more mileage out of our marriage and our intimate physical life. She referred me to a physical therapist and a hypnotist, who also gave me a lot of help. The hypnotist even helped me stop smoking! I'd have to say that this group kind of saved our lives. They're not all great, I'm told, but this one really was.

Ralph: We got some good help from a shrink when I was first diagnosed. The problem was I couldn't get hard—my penis. I couldn't get an erection, and it just about did me in. Right away, one day, bang! I was impotent and it wrecked me for a while. My wife dragged me off to some group therapy and self-help kind of groups. I was embarrassed to talk in them so I told her I'd prefer a one-on-one session with a shrink, either a psychologist or therapist. I wasn't exactly sure of the difference, if there is one. We worked with this guy for a few months, and he saw me—us—through a lot of screaming and yelling on my part. He helped me to stop feeling sorry for myself, which was a bigger problem than I realized, and helped both of us come to terms with the situation, and get a lot more self-esteem, both of us, and to figure out ways we could salvage what was left of our sex life. As it turned out, my problem was only a temporary thing that tended to come and go, so it wasn't as bad as I first thought. Still, the therapist helped us a lot.

DEALING WITH ANGER, DEPRESSION, AND FEAR

Perhaps the three most common negative feelings patients with multiple sclerosis experience are anger, depression, and fear. Occasionally these emotions are produced by the pathology of the disease itself and by its effects on the limbic system of the brain, where most of our emotions originate. More frequently, they are a response to the anxieties it produces.

Although anger, depression, and fear tend to be especially common immediately after a diagnosis of MS is received, they sometimes linger on for months and even years, popping up spontaneously and uninvited to cloud the already cloudy waters. Several MS patients talk about the persistence of these emotions:

- "Every morning when I wake up and realize my legs don't work right I go through a kind of mini-anger tantrum deep inside myself. It happens every day like clockwork."

- "As time passes I'll be feeling better. Then boom! I'll get depressed thinking that I'll not be the same as I was before I got sick. The struggle with depression continues on. It's something you have to keep dealing with all the time."

- "I've had MS for years. I still have to fight off the despair and loss of self-esteem it brings. The embarrassment of not being able to hold a pencil right—you don't walk correctly. Even though my condition has stabilized, the very thought of it coming back makes me feel frightened a lot of the time and full of worry."

• "It's the anger that kills you. Anger. You want to punch your pillow or the wall and . . . you want to scream and yell at the top of your lungs. But you know that if you do it too long and hard you'll get exhausted and have to sit down and pant for a while to get your breath back. So you see, you don't even have the luxury of getting mad at life without feeling sick and overtired. You're not even allowed that simple pleasure . . . and that in itself makes me mad."

Depression is probably the most common form of anguish among MS patients, and the most enduring. It affects 40 to 50 percent of the MS population, and is particularly common during periods of exacerbation.

Here a word of explanation is in order, for when discussing clinical depression many misconceptions arise, the most prevalent being that depression is simply an intensification of feeling "down" or "blue." In some cases, of course, MS persons do indeed report prolonged bouts of melancholy and tears. Others, however, live through depression without experiencing any sensations of sadness or dejection per se. Instead, they undergo what are called *neuro-vegetative* symptoms, palpable physical complaints that affect persons in a variety of seemingly unconnected ways. Typical examples include insomnia, early-morning awakenings, constipation, changes in appetite and weight, reduction in sexual interest, memory deficits, lack of concentration, flattening of emotional affect, and overall fatigue and lack of energy.

At the heart of depression stands a fundamental cause: *loss.* In the case of an MS patient, this loss is not only of body function, not only of the normal pleasures of living we all take so for granted, but of future possibilities in the social, business, and personal realms of life as well. And since multiple sclerosis is primarily a disease of youth, such loss is especially bitter to the young men and women who are starting out in marriage or on a job, and who it seemed just yesterday had the world at their feet.

"I've been conned by life," one young MS patient remarks. "Robbed of my inheritance—the right to lead a happy life with a body that's working okay and is still intact."

No wonder then that dark, anguished emotions of one sort or another creep in. How could they not?

At the same time, while such feelings are inevitable and per-haps even therapeutic in the beginning, over the long haul they tend to become counterproductive. At times they turn undeniably self-destructive.

What can be done to deal with the emotional ups and downs that MS persons experience? What methods exist for channeling the negatives into positives, and for reducing the psychological burden that so many MS patients are forced to shoulder? There are a variety of possible answers. Let's have a look at some of the most helpful.

ATTITUDE IS EVERYTHING

Feelings of fear, worry, anxiety, despair, and frustration are emo-tional responses triggered by real and present dangers outside oneself. Of this there is no doubt. From another perspective, however, these feelings originate and are generated entirely *inside one's own mind*.

Looking at things from this standpoint, mental and emotional reactions are ultimately self-generated, and hence in many cases controllable as well. There is, after all, not a lot patients can do about the fact that they have MS. They had no say concerning their getting it, and they can do nothing to make it go away. There are, however, critical things they *can* do to control their mental reactions to having this disease and to adapting to their new life circumstances, and herein lies the key. Note the following steps you can take to form a confident attitude and to overcome the negative "debris" that tends to plague the lives of persons with MS:

1. *Start by being as honest with yourself as you can.*

You have the disease. This is a reality. And unless a wonder cure appears sometime soon, things are probably going to remain this way.

So avoid denial. Avoid buoying yourself up with false expectations. Look the matter straight in the eye: you have multiple sclerosis. This is the situation, and this is probably the way it is going to remain for years to come. Face this fact as best you can.

2. *Enumerate the positives.*

After coming to terms with this difficult reality, realize next that there are a number of mitigating and even potentially positive elements to the situation. For example:

• Many MS patients experience mild symptoms only. Some have a flareup or two and then never undergo symptoms of any kind.

• MS is an unpredictable disease that cannot be second-guessed. You therefore have two choices: either imagine the worst or imagine the best. If you imagine the worst, you will be plagued by anger, depression, and fear. If you dwell on the best, hope will prevail. So why not imagine the best? It feels better that way, and it's better for you. All in all, moreover, the statistics are on your side.

• When people first discover they have MS they sometimes become preoccupied with secret thoughts of suicide; this, in fact, is a frequent response to a serious medical diagnosis of any kind. Yet although suicidal ideations among MS patients tend to be common, especially in the early stages, actual rates of self-inflicted death are surprisingly low, comprising less than 1 percent of the MS population. Why? Because after the initial shock of discovery, patients discover that MS is a manageable disease and that life really does go on after diagnosis. The world around us is filled with thousands and thousands of MS persons who were once ready to give up on it all, but who are now leading adjusted, productive lives.

• Although MS produces many difficult symptoms, in most cases medications and therapeutic techniques exist that will keep them under control. Again remember: MS is a manageable disease.

• There are many other persons like you in this country today, persons who have MS and who are anxious to share their experience and know-how with others. Mutual support goes a long way and can be a tremendous consolation for persons who are feeling overwhelmed. More information on self-help and community support groups will be provided at the end of this section.

3. *Develop a positive attitude.*

Keep telling yourself that a positive attitude really does count, and that the less you dwell on the negatives the more pleasant and manageable life will become.

Don't underestimate the power of such inner dialogue. All of us are conditioned by the positive and negative things we tell ourselves every day. Confidence, self-assurance, security, strength of will—and on the other side, fear, frustration, anxiety, lack of confidence—all are born of the ideas we hourly invite into our heads, and of the words we repeat to ourselves as we pass through the course of a day.

If one's thinking is affirmative and one dwells on the things that can be done and not on the things that cannot be undone, one's life will follow suit; if not, one must be prepared to suffer the consequences. In this sense, we all possess the power to control our own mental and emotional destinies no matter how bad things seem to be in the external world. We have only to make the effort.

4. *Be of service to others.*

One of the best, though largely unheralded, antidotes to depression is service to other people. Participating in charitable enterprises, doing volunteer work, working with the underprivileged, helping one's friends and neighbors in times of need, joining community or church groups—these activities produce a kind of therapeutic effect on persons that is difficult to measure but that is very real to those who experience it. Just ask them:

Sid R.: As far as the things I did to overcome feeling lousy about the MS, the best thing was the Rotary Club service I performed, and continuing to work with the kids in the Babe Ruth League. I'd be feeling really down and wouldn't want to even go out of the house. Then the kids come by and say "Let's go, Sid old Kid." I'd hobble out with my cane and join them on the ball field for a few hours, shouting out advice and manager talk from the sideline and sometimes pitching batting practice when I was up to it. In the middle of it all I would almost always stop for a minute and think to myself how much better I felt now that I was here working with the kids and having so much fun, and seeing them have fun too.

Nancy R.: Both my parents suggested that I do some volunteer work in the neighborhood. I was lying around the house feeling sorry for myself. "Get up and get out there and help someone," my mother said to me. "It will make you feel better." I worked in a hospital for a time. I would get real tired and couldn't work long hours, but they were appreciative and asked me back, and that made my self-esteem soar. Now I work in our local National Multiple Sclerosis office as a volunteer several days a week and it makes me feel good about myself too. Helping others, I've found, is kind of like the same thing as helping yourself.

Rose L.: I've felt the best when I've been out of the house helping my daughter take care of her two children. If you want my recipe for feeling good it's this: Go out and help others. It doesn't matter who. It will help you forget your own problems no matter how serious they are. In my case—and you don't have to believe this if you don't want to—it's made me grateful for my life, even though I'm in a wheelchair. Yes, I said grateful. Feeling grateful stops you from feeling sorry for yourself and alone. Feeling grateful makes you feel better than eating a chocolate ice cream cone or having sex. That's right, better than both of these things. I strongly recommend helping others and feeling grateful as a way of conquering multiple sclerosis. I know of what I speak, believe me.

5. *Aim for acceptance.*

It is a well-known psychological fact that when a personal difficulty is accepted and integrated into the activities of ordinary behavior it ceases to exert a negative grip and becomes a neutral fact of life that persons deal with as best they can within the context of normal living.

But how, it might be asked, does one learn to accept a difficulty as truly burdensome as MS?

By following the instructions given above. By accentuating the positive and "decentuating" the negative. By rejecting hopeless thoughts and emphasizing hopeful ones. By remaining active and involved in the activities that interest you. And by making conscious mental efforts whenever possible to strive toward a state of acceptance. "I tell myself over and over," one patient reports, "that I have this disease in my spine and brain, that it's here to stay. I have to make the best of it. I have to keep going and take care of the household and the children and my home business. I tell this to myself over and over. I'm getting to the point where I can live with what's happening to me now, and build my life around it. There's peace for me in that."

What exactly does acceptance mean? Acceptance is an intuition of sorts, a kind of global assumption patients make that they will somehow survive whatever comes their way, and that it's all right to go on living and working and plowing ahead as best they can, even though they know that at times the going will be rough. "Hope," as the Jewish scholar Avery Weisman once remarked, "means that we have confidence in the *desirability* of survival."

Patients will recognize acceptance in themselves when they no longer spend inordinate amounts of time thinking about their disease or dwelling on its negative effects. Also:

• When they find themselves worrying less about the consequences of the disease and about how it will affect them tomorrow and the day after.

• When they see MS as just another part of their lives and not the central core.

• When they are able to make the appropriate adjustments to their symptoms and to the changing life circumstances that MS brings.

• When they live more in the present and spend less time dwelling on the future and the past.

• When they admit to themselves that they have MS and do not become immediately frightened.

• When they can face the possibility that their disease may become worse and still not panic.

• When they experience an open willingness—or at least a bottom-line acquiescence—to accept whatever it is that fate may now bring.

Acceptance, one might say, is an attitude of optimistic resignation.

Another way acceptance can be recognized is when an MS person ceases to dwell on unreasonable expectations. This is true for persons with all degrees of disabilities, from transient vision problems to permanent loss of ambulation. Yes, patients tell themselves, I may be experiencing certain serious symptoms; yes, I will be looked at somewhat differently by my family and friends and coworkers from now on; and no, they tell themselves, I will not be able to do all the things I did before I was sick; and no, I cannot tell what the future will bring. Yet I accept this situation as best I can. It is not, after all, the end of the world. I do not wish to prolong my sadness and mourning more than necessary; this would be counterproductive. Life goes on, and I have the right to live it as fully as I can. I have my mind and feelings, my family, my friends, my job, my interests, my goals, my life. For me this is now enough.

In general, it is known that persons who deal best with MS on a psychological level are those who plunge into life no matter how disabled they may be. Such persons take an active interest in their own medical care. They work hard to maintain their health, their mental acuity, their relationships and family life. They avoid feelings of self-pity as best they can, and strive to remain socially available and attentive to other people's feelings and needs. They remain, in short, active, involved, and alive.

Such people know how to set limits on their own energies, and how to budget their time. They cultivate methods for getting the most out of whatever it is they are doing—how to prioritize daily chores, how to put aside worry for the future and extract the best from things *right now*. Hobbies, entertainments, romance, sports, friendships, learning, intellectual pursuits, religious faith, living one's life to its fullest sense of purpose are all forms of medication against the doldrums that MS brings. If, after going through the down times, a person wakes up one morning and feels that, yes, I am alive, and that, yes, I do want to continue on, and that, yes, I *can* continue to live an active, productive life, all this is good evidence that a state of acceptance is within that person's reach, and that the psychological self-healing process is under way.

MEDICATION AND DEPRESSION

During those moments when depression and emotional distress become especially intense, an antidepressant medication may be the therapy of choice. Physicians, however, are not always in agreement on this point. Some insist that at the first sign of mental distress a patient should immediately be given the option of taking antidepressant or tranquilizing medications. Others believe that emotions such as depression and anger are the mind's natural way of working through its problems, and that to tamper with this self-regulating mechanism by prescribing chemical palliatives is to sabotage a process that will ultimately produce important healing effects.

When, then, it could be asked, are antidepressant medications appropriate and necessary?

The only rules-of-thumb here are the ones patients set for themselves. That is, when and if a person feels overwhelmed by mental distress and has the need for relief, by all means that person should ask for medication. Neurologists are well versed in antidepressant drugs and know which varieties are appropriate for the situation at hand. Although these drugs will not provide total freedom from anxiety, and though they certainly will not cure the underlying problems, they take enough edge off the pain to allow patients to return to a relatively normal daily existence.

Some patients, it should be mentioned, are reluctant to request antidepressant medication for fear that their doctor and friends will view them as "crazy" or as "mentally disturbed." But surely this is a false and dangerous fear. The psychological mood disturbances that multiple sclerosis may cause are sometimes profound, more profound than a person can handle at times, and when this condition occurs patients are urged to seek help in whatever form is available. To repress one's anxiety and say nothing about it is to make matters worse, not better, like trying to prevent a pot from boiling by pushing down on its lid. "Unfortunately, some MSers are unwilling to take antidepressant medications because of the social stigma of any 'psychiatric' diagnosis," writes Dr. John K. Wolf. "If you recognize yourself in this chapter but have that lingering prejudice, please re-think your priorities. Are you more interested in avoiding the diagnosis of a treatable symptom of MS than in returning to your life?"*

What type of drugs are most often prescribed for depression? The star of the field these days is the tricyclic family of antidepressants, especially Elavil (chemical name, amitriptyline) and Tofranil (imipramine). These preparations usually come in tablet, capsule, or syrup form, are not habit-forming, and tend to work impressively well with a wide range of patients.

Except in extreme cases, moreover, the side effects of a typical tricyclic such as Elavil or Tofranil are relatively benign. They include headache, dry mouth, drowsiness, indigestion, bowel problems, extreme sweating, and sometimes nausea. In rare instances, tremor, insomnia, glaucoma, hallucinations, and extreme

---

*John K. Wolf, M.D., et al., *Mastering Multiple Sclerosis: A Guide to Management*. Rutland, Vermont: Academy Books, 1987.

fatigue will result, in which case the drug should be discontinued and the issue discussed with a physician. Users of Elavil and tricyclic drugs in general should, however, be careful of mixing the drug with alcohol or of using it with antihistamines, barbiturates, and anticoagulants. Since the tricyclics tend to make users drowsy, it is recommended that these medications be taken at night immediately before going to sleep.

Another fact to realize about the tricyclics is that they take time to build up an effective blood level and to work at maximum capacity. Two or three weeks is the average time for the medication to start taking effect; in some cases a month to six weeks will be required. During this period a person may continue to be depressed and may assume that the drug is not doing its job. But this is not necessarily the case; it may simply be a matter of waiting it out a week or two longer before the effects kick in.

Antidepressants are often prescribed for limited periods of time, say six months to a year, and then discontinued. In some instances the depression will then be gone and will not return. In other cases, further medication may be required. This is not a cause for worry, however, as few serious long-term effects of tricyclic drugs have been reported.

While antidepressants are by far the most common medications prescribed for mental upset and mood swings, other drugs may work better in certain cases. Tranquilizers such as Valium and Xanax will relax anxious patients and reduce the intensity of their fears. Levodopa, a drug commonly given to Parkinson's patients for controlling rigidity and bradykinesia, is sometimes prescribed for MS patients who are prone to rages and emotional outbursts. For patients with sleep difficulties, sedatives are sometimes in order. Other commonly used antidepressant medications besides Elavil and Tofranil include Adapin and Sinequan (chemical name, doxepin), and Presamine and Imavate (imipramine). All are effective potions, and the choice of one over the other is a matter of physician preference.

Finally, if an MS patient is pregnant, has recently undergone surgery, suffers from heart disease, hypertension, or allergies, he or she must be certain to report these matters to the physician before beginning a course of antidepressants, or any other form of psychotropic medications.

ALTERNATE METHODS FOR COMBATING NEGATIVITY AND DEPRESSION

Here are some grassroots tips for overcoming depression and negative emotions that patients have reported through the years. Many of the methods are hit-or-miss and anecdotal; that is, they work for some persons and not for others. All are harmless and are commonly recommended by counselors and medical professionals. Test them if you feel so inclined; many patients speak highly in their favor.

• *Try vitamins*—There is much anecdotal lore concerning the antidepressant value of certain vitamins, minerals, and food supplements. Most doctors will tell you that nothing substantial has been clinically established concerning the positive effects of these items on depression and stress. Nonetheless, many MS patients swear by them. You be the judge.

The following supplements have at one time or another been put forward as useful against depression, anxiety, and stress.

Calcium or calcium lactate—a reputed specific for depression, anxiety, and stress. Approximately 250 to 500 mgs a day (or more) is recommended. Some physicians believe it's best to take these pills at night before you go to bed, as much of the body's calcium metabolism takes place while we sleep.

B-Complex—Recommended for anxiety, nervousness, and stress (vitamin B has been called the "nerve vitamin"). Specifics for stress include B_1 (thiamine), B_6 (pyridoxine), and pantothenic acid, all of which can be found in a good B-complex vitamin. Niacin is sometimes recommended by nutritionists for insomnia caused by stress.

Vitamin D—Occasionally recommended for stress.

L-Tyrosine—An amino acid said to be useful for combating chronic depression. Take 500 mgs a day for several weeks and see if it helps.

Vitamin C—Simply a good all-round vitamin supplement to have on the medicine shelf and one touted by some as helping depression. Take 500 mgs a day, and supplement it with plenty of leafy greens, citrus fruits, and fruit juices.

Sunflower seed oil (linoleic)—An essential fatty acid said to help depression.

• *Get better organized*—Feeling overwhelmed by the demands made by family, job, social life, and economic concerns can sometimes become a major cause of anxiety. Postponed telephone calls, letters not written, beds not made, bills not paid, groceries not purchased, obligations not met, untidy rooms, messy desks, unfulfilled promises, all exert a subtle but decidedly stressful effect on a person's day.

Getting organized can help. Write it down in a notebook. Pin it up on the wall. Keep it on file in plain view. Compile check lists, date books, calendars, schedules. Start the morning by reviewing the day's obligations, then methodically fulfill these obligations one by one. Know your limits. Take on a single task at a time and don't try to juggle too many balls at once. Choose your priorities carefully and guard against procrastination. Most of all, don't be afraid to say no when you're in over your head—the first axiom of getting organized is not to bite off more than you can chew.

• *Get enough rest and sleep*—Sounds simple enough. But for many MS persons burning the candle at both ends can do more than simply overtire; it can sap one's fundamental store of energy to the core, leaving one tense, nervous, and depleted.

Don't, moreover, make the mistake of thinking that because you used to get along with seven hours of sleep at night before the MS appeared the same situation still applies. In many cases, MS persons will need considerably more rest during the day and sleep at night than the ordinary person; stinting in this department can often get one in trouble.

• *Be sure to exercise*—Exercise has been discussed at length throughout this book, and for good reason: it is a specific not only against stiffness but in some cases for fatigue and depression as well. "Exercise is well-known to be crucial to staying emotionally as well as physically healthy," claims a tract on the subject of emotional adjustment published by the National Multiple Sclerosis Society. "And this applies to the person with MS as much as to anyone else. An exercise regimen tailored to your condition can be beneficial in the treatment of depression and anxiety. Recent studies of the chemical effects of exercise on the brain, show that regular, somewhat vigorous exercise can release chemicals called endorphins into the brain, having some of the same effects as tranquilizers, muscle relaxants, and sedatives. Another study found a positive relationship between exercise and both mood and one's thinking process."*

Patients who suffer emotional ups and downs and who are fit enough to exercise will find that a daily course of stretching and aerobics will relieve inner tensions and reduce the general level of stress and worry. Consult Chapter 6 for the specifics.

• *Practice relaxation techniques*—Muscular tensions and knots, often unfelt and undetected on a conscious level, exist throughout our joint and muscular systems. These tensions exert low-level internal pressures that over time sap energy and create sensations of mental heaviness and physical discomfort. For some persons an effective antidote is formal relaxation technique.

Chapter 7 offers several such techniques. Another exercise, which can be practiced whenever one has a few leisure minutes and which is especially useful for anxiety and depression, is as follows:

Lie or sit in a relaxed position. Close your eyes and loosen your clothing. Take a deep breath and let it out slowly. With each inhalation say to yourself "I am." With each exhalation say "relaxed."

Continue to repeat this sentence to yourself subverbally and

*Mary Sanford, Ph.D, and Jack Petajan, M.D., *Multiple Sclerosis and Your Emotions*. New York, Multiple Sclerosis Society, 1989.

form a picture in your mind's eye of the most pleasant scene you can imagine. It may be the beach, a forest, a breath-taking panorama.

Contemplate this image for several minutes, then walk into it. If you are looking at a mountain landscape, enter the landscape. Stroll through the meadows. Pick a wildflower and feel it in your hands. Experience the mountain air on the back of your neck. Listen to a nearby brook. Dwell in this wonderland as long as you like, all the while repeating "I am—relaxed."

When finished, gently dissolve the picture, take a deep breath, and open your eyes. By now you should be thoroughly relaxed.

• *Meditate*—For some MS persons, taking a half-hour out of the day for quiet sitting and concentration on such points of attention as one's breath, an inspirational idea, a poem, a mantra, or a prayer has a calming, centering effect that, some believe, cannot be duplicated by other forms of relaxation.

Many books on medication technique can be found in bookstores, and religious and philosophical organizations of both Eastern and Western persuasion are located in most parts of the country today. Check the newspaper or the listings on local community bulletin boards for information.

• *Take care of your psychic needs*—Find a quiet place for yourself and visit it frequently. Tests have shown that stress levels are dramatically reduced when persons schedule a fixed amount of time from the day to simply sit down, relax, and let go.

When you feel the urge, cry. Crying is a fine way to relieve anxiety and to reduce psychological strain. When persons hold back tears they hold in tension. It is not by accident that human beings are the only animals that have tear ducts.

Develop a hobby. Outside interests are classic stress reducers. It doesn't matter what the hobby is: model ships, needlepoint, cooking, stamp collecting, computers, painting, cabinetmaking, poetry, a foreign language. The point is to find a recreational activity that is physically or mentally absorbing and then pursue it.

Share your problems. Talk to other people: friends, family,

people who care and whose advice you value. Talking to sympathetic others can at times have a kind of magical effect, defusing the tension and reducing inner pressures. It's the safety-valve principle at work: let off some of the steam and the internal pressure won't become too great.

• *Seek professional and support-group help*—Not knowing when the next flareup is coming, or how quickly one's symptoms will progress, or realizing that the disease is incurable can all exert long-term wearing effects on a person's nerves. During acute exacerbations, fear and confusion levels escalate dramatically, putting a person into a psychological crisis that may require expert guidance and medications to control. Then, when the flareup passes, a negative psychic aftermath sometimes remains, with disorientation continuing for weeks and even months after the symptoms themselves have disappeared.

Receiving a diagnosis of MS can send a person into a state of emotional distress. As the reality of the new situation sinks in and physical discomfort increases, the MS person becomes more in need of sympathy from family and friends than ever before, and at the same time becomes more needy and demanding. Family members burdened with caregiving pressures for long periods of time may finally lose patience with the sick person's complaints. Since so many symptoms of MS are fluctuating and invisible, the patient's vague claims of fatigue or blurry vision arouse skepticism and thoughts of hypochondria in family members. Physical pain and emotional uncertainty add to the complications; the more patients suffer the more alone and misunderstood they feel. In response, they lash out at others around them, alienating friends and family members who once stood by faithfully, ready to help. Eventually this vicious circle spins an entire family into a void of hostility, alienation, and separation. Divorce rates among MS patients are considerably higher than the average.

It is therefore not unusual for MS patients in crisis to be referred to a mental-health professional or group-support system of some kind. Psychiatrists, psychologists, family counselors, social workers, group-therapy leaders, self-help organizations, and therapists of many degrees of expertise are all available.

In many cases, for example, short-term counseling—a few weeks to a year—is all that is needed to get a person back on track. Individual counseling focuses on whatever needs the patient brings to the session: the need for guidance while working through reactions to diagnosis or progressive flareups, for instance, or helping a person get a grip when the circumstances of life seem too great to bear are typical matters for therapeutic discussion. For persons with deeper and older problems made worse by the knowledge that they have MS, long-term counseling or psychotherapy is also available. During such sessions therapists will concentrate on delving below the surface of a patient's transient anxieties into the deeper causes that underlie the neurosis.

Group-therapy sessions and support groups sponsored by such organizations as the National Multiple Sclerosis Society are another popular option. When first meeting with other MS sufferers and discussing the thorny issues caused by MS, patients are often surprised, then gratified, to learn that other people face the same problems as themselves, and that no sufferer from MS need suffer alone.

During group meetings much information of a practical and psychological nature is traded. Attendees at a typical gathering of a National Multiple Sclerosis support group, for example, might air a spectrum of concerns ranging from the best way to clean a catheter to sources for buying ankle braces, from recent books on the subject of MS to the best way to apply for government benefits. Other patients, it turns out, have, like oneself, experienced a variety of bowel and urinary embarrassments, and have come up with ingenious ways for solving them, which they gladly share with others. "Unmentionable" topics such as incontinence or impotence or thoughts of suicide, suddenly become less threatening when brought up and out for group discussion. Indeed, in many support groups patients literally find themselves joking about personal issues that yesterday they might not have mentioned to their best friend.

Group discussion is a useful social as well as psychological tool. New friendships are made at these meetings, and mutual support networks are established, in which members keep in close personal touch or maintain daily telephone contact in case of emergency. For many persons the simple act of gathering once or twice a week with a group of like-minded associates under the guidance of a trained and sympathetic leader can exert a healing influence that goes a long way toward returning one to emotional stability. A family physician, neurologist, local hospital, the National Multiple Sclerosis Foundation main offices in New York City (see Appendix for address), one of the 150 local chapters of the NMSS, and/or members of any local MS support group whatever its affiliation are all potential sources of referrals and recommendations for individual therapy, group therapy, and/or support-group meetings.

• *Develop an inner life*—Finally, there is the question of gaining psychological and emotional strength through the development of a spiritual inner life. For when all is said and done, MS persons have only their bodies and their hearts to get them through this long, difficult trial. Their bodies will more or less serve them at the task, even if they are slowed down a bit by demyelinating disease. Their psychic parts, on the other hand, their secret selves, are more delicate and vulnerable; these parts must be nurtured now with special sensitivity if patients are to experience the full range of joy, awareness, and transcendence that belongs to all men and to all women as part of their human inheritance. Though each MS patient is different, vast numbers have drawn their greatest strength from this understanding: that beneath all human exteriors lies a single common need for the eternal verities—patience, contentment, worship, and something permanent beyond the material world.

Thus, while each MS person must seek his or her own God, each person *needs* to seek. Without an aspiration for something beyond the trivialities of the TV set and the marketplace, we grow cynical and weary, and the health of the body declines along with the spirit. If our goal is indeed to make the most of our condition, whatever it happens to be—today, tomorrow, and the day after that—then we must find a set of beliefs that benefit the whole man, the whole woman, and we must cleave to it.

For as humankind has known from time beginning, the search for *real* health, for health of the soul and the heart as well as of the muscle and blood, inevitably begins—and ends—within.

Appendix

Medical Mail-Order Sources

Note: All the following companies issue extensive catalogs. Inquire directly.

Abbey Medical
17390 Brookhurst Street
Suite 200
Fountain Valley, California 92708

Arthritis Self-Help Products
3 Little Knoll Court
Medford, New Jersey 08055

Cleo, Inc.
3957 Mayfield Road
Cleveland, Ohio 44121

Enrichments
145 Tower Drive
P.O. Box 579
Hinsdale, Illinois 60521

Fred Sammons
P.O. Box 32
Brookfield, Illinois 60513

HSA Health Suppliers
P.O. Box 288
Farmville, North Carolina 27828

Mature Wisdom
Hanover, Pennsylvania 17333

Products for People with Vision Problems
Consumer Products
American Foundation for the Blind
15 West 16th Street
New York, New York 10011

Selected Bibliography

The following are helpful books on MS and related subjects:

Lechtenberg, Richard, *Multiple Sclerosis Fact Book*. Philadelphia, PA, Davis Company, 1988

Maloff, Chalda, and Susan Macduff Wood, *Business and Social Etiquette with Disabled People*. Springfield, IL, Charles C. Thomas, 1988.

Matthews, Bryan, *Multiple Sclerosis: The Facts*. New York, Oxford University Press, 1985.

Perkins, Lanny, and Sara Perkins, *Multiple Sclerosis: Your Legal Rights*. New York, Demos Publications, 1988.

Petajan, J.H., ed., *Multiple Sclerosis Handbook*. Salt Lake City, UT, National Multiple Sclerosis Society, Utah Chapter, 1980.

Rosner, Louis, and Shelley Ross, *Multiple Sclerosis: New Hope and Practical Advice*. Old Tappan, NJ, Prentice Hall Press, 1987.

Schapiro, Randall, *Multiple Sclerosis: A Rehabilitation Approach to Management*. New York, Demos Publications, 1991.

———, *System Management in Multiple Sclerosis*. New York, Demos Publications, 1987.

Scheinberg, Labe, and Nancy Holland, eds., *Multiple Sclerosis: A Guide for Patients and Their Families*. New York, Raven Press, 1987, second edition.

Shuman, Robert, and Janica Schwartz, *Understanding Multiple Sclerosis: A New Handbook for Families*. New York, Charles Scribner's Sons, 1988.

Sibley, William, *Therapeutic Claims in Multiple Sclerosis*. New York, Demos Publications, 1988, second edition.

Strong, Maggie, *Mainstay: For the Well Spouse of the Chronically Ill*. Boston, Little Brown, 1988.

Waksman, B.H., and S.C. Reingold, *Research on Multiple Sclerosis*. New York, Demos Publications, 1988.

Wolf, John K. (with others), *Mastering Multiple Sclerosis: A Guide to Management*. Rutland, VT, Academy Books, 1987, second edition.

———— (with others), *Fall Down Seven Times Get Up Eight: Living Hell with Multiple Sclerosis*. Rutland, VT, Academy Books, 1991.

See also all publications from the National Multiple Sclerosis Society, 733 Third Avenue, New York, NY 10017. Many of these are free, and all are valuable. Free copies of *Inside Magazine*—especially for MS patients and their families—may be obtained by writing to the MS Society.

Index